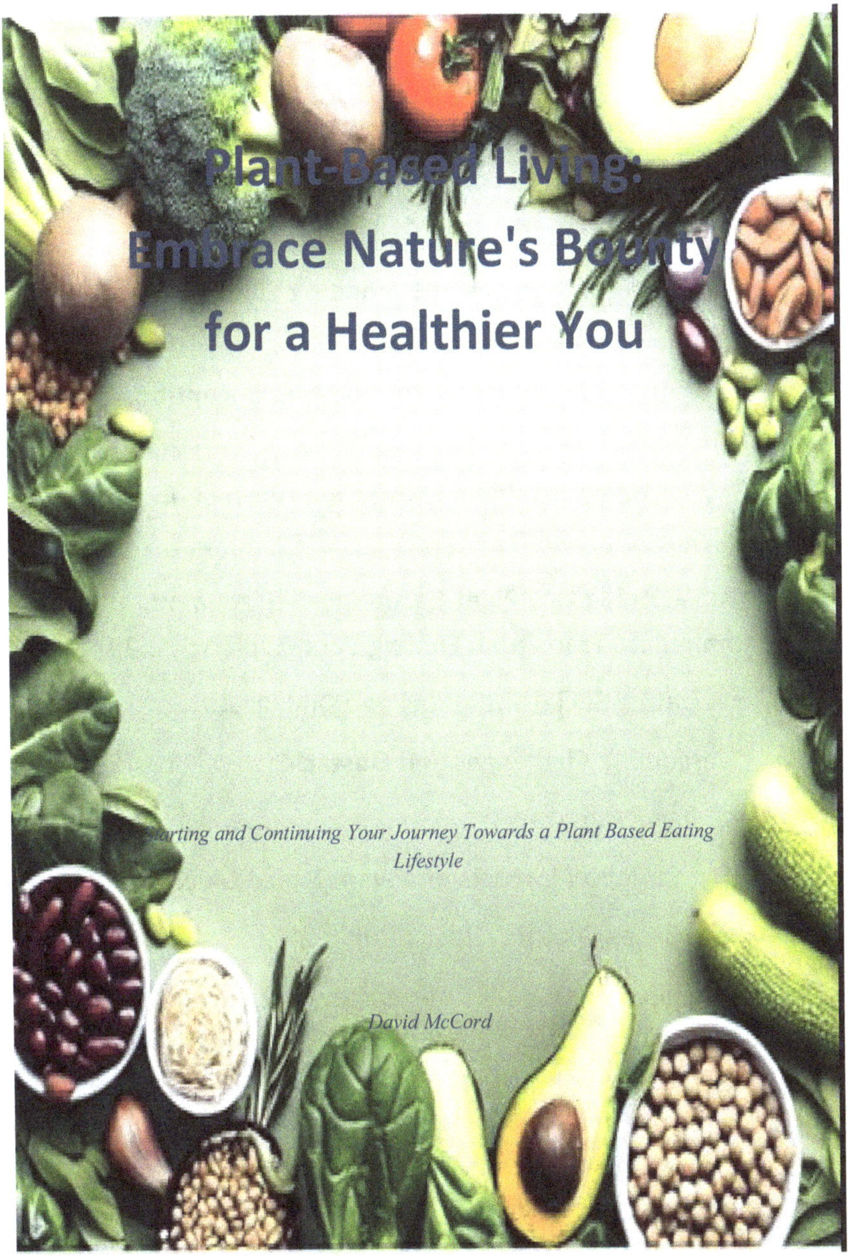

Plant-Based Living: Embrace Nature's Bounty for a Healthier You

Starting and Continuing Your Journey Towards a Plant Based Eating Lifestyle

David McCord

Table of Contents:

Contents

Introduction:

Welcome to "Plant-Based Living: Embrace Nature's Bounty for a Healthier You!" In this comprehensive book/e-book, we embark on a journey that celebrates the incredible power of plants and how they can transform our lives for the better. Whether you are already a plant-based enthusiast or just beginning to explore this lifestyle, this guide is designed to empower and inspire you to embrace the nourishing and compassionate path of plant-based living.

The world is witnessing a growing awareness of the impact our dietary choices have on our health, the environment, and the well-being of animals.

With this newfound awareness, the plant-based movement has gained momentum, appealing to individuals seeking a healthier, more sustainable, and compassionate way of life. A plant-based diet centers around consuming foods primarily derived from plants, including vegetables, fruits, grains, legumes, nuts, and seeds, while minimizing or eliminating animal-derived products.

In this book/e-book, we'll delve into the numerous benefits of adopting a plant-based lifestyle. We'll explore the abundance of essential nutrients available in plant-based foods, dispel common myths and misconceptions,

and provide practical tips to help you transition seamlessly into this rewarding way of eating. Whether you're seeking to enhance your well-being, lose weight, manage chronic conditions, or simply feel more energized and vibrant, a well-planned plant-based diet can be your key to achieving these goals.

We understand that transitioning to a plant-based diet may seem overwhelming at first, but fear not! Throughout the following chapters, we'll guide you step-by-step, offering advice on meal planning, essential kitchen tools, and delicious plant-based alternatives for your favorite dishes.

You'll discover that plant-based cooking is not only easy and enjoyable but also a gateway to a world of diverse flavors and culinary creativity.

Beyond personal health benefits, our plant-based journey extends to the welfare of our planet. We'll explore how plant-based living aligns with sustainable practices and reduces our environmental footprint.

Embracing a plant-based diet is a powerful way to contribute to a greener and more sustainable future for generations to come.

This book/e-book is intended to be a comprehensive resource for all aspects of plant-based living.

From breakfast delights to hearty lunches, delectable dinners to sweet treats, we'll present a plethora of recipes that showcase the incredible variety and deliciousness of plant-based foods. Moreover, we'll address the nutritional concerns that some may have and provide guidance on maintaining a balanced and thriving plant-based diet.

Whether you're a curious beginner, a seasoned plant-based enthusiast, or someone looking to make a positive change in their life, this book/e-book will equip you with the knowledge and tools you need to embark on your plant-based journey confidently.

Our goal is to empower you to embrace the transformative power of plants and witness the positive impact they can have on your well-being and the world around you.

So, let's begin this exciting adventure together as we embrace the beauty and nourishment that plant-based living has to offer. Get ready to

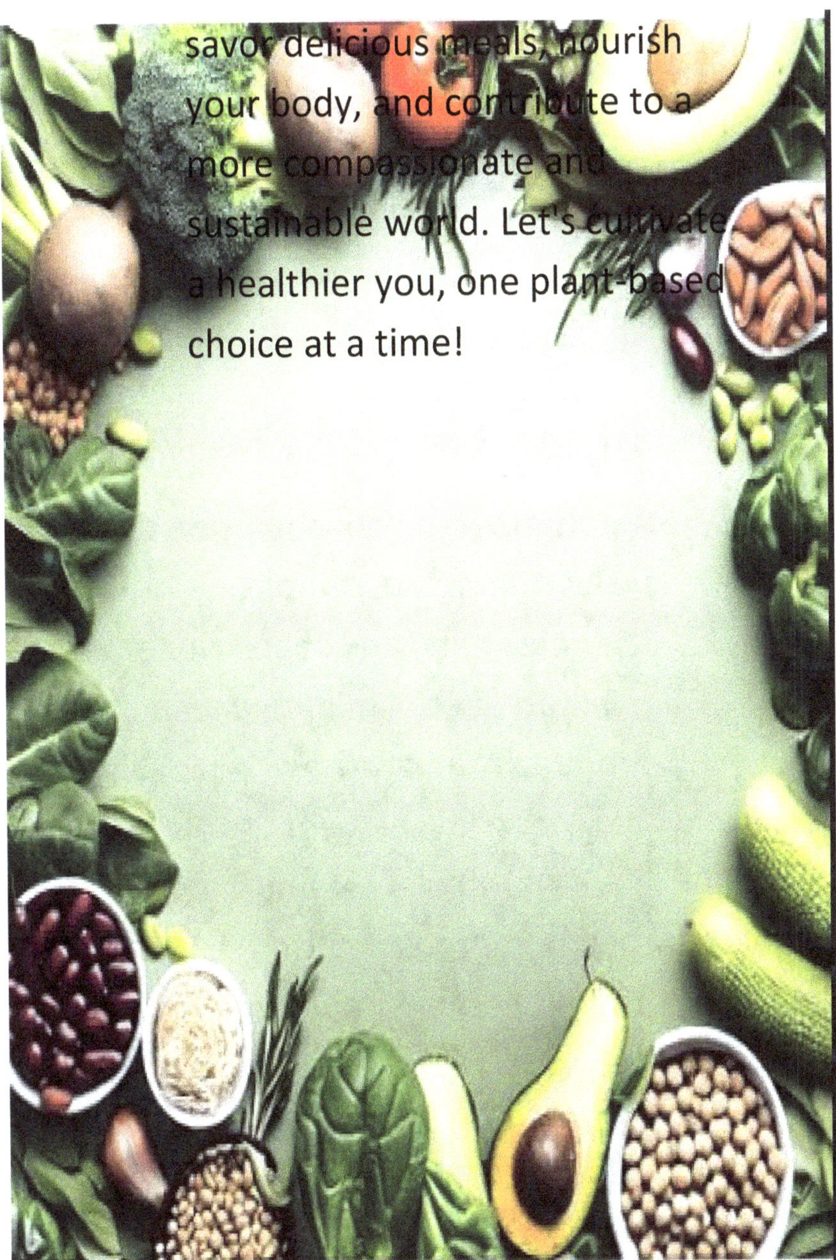
savor delicious meals, nourish your body, and contribute to a more compassionate and sustainable world. Let's cultivate a healthier you, one plant-based choice at a time!

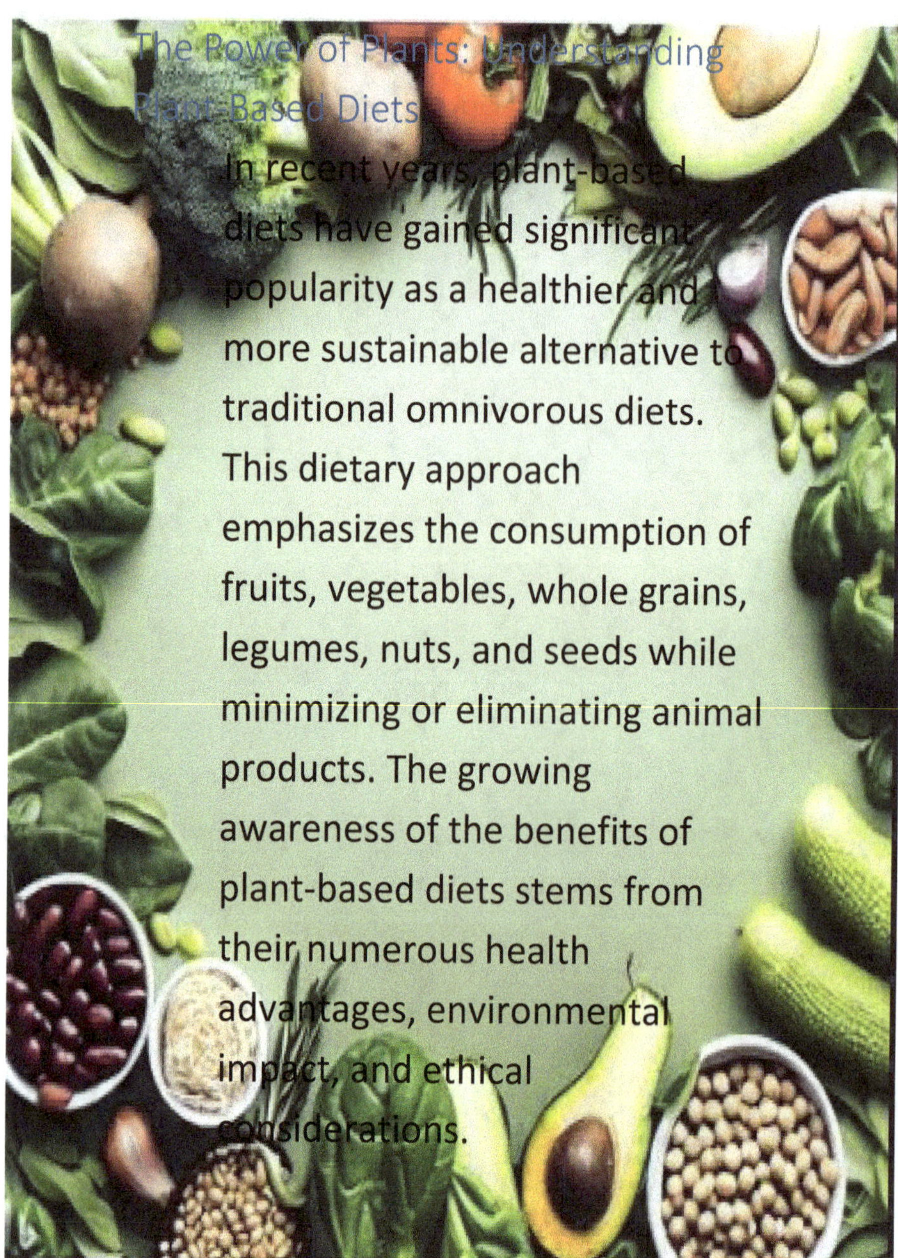

The Power of Plants: Understanding Plant-Based Diets

In recent years, plant-based diets have gained significant popularity as a healthier and more sustainable alternative to traditional omnivorous diets. This dietary approach emphasizes the consumption of fruits, vegetables, whole grains, legumes, nuts, and seeds while minimizing or eliminating animal products. The growing awareness of the benefits of plant-based diets stems from their numerous health advantages, environmental impact, and ethical considerations.

One of the most compelling reasons people adopt plant-based diets is the positive impact on overall health. Research has shown that plant-based diets can reduce the risk of chronic diseases such as heart disease, diabetes, obesity, and certain types of cancer. The abundance of essential vitamins, minerals, and antioxidants in plant-based foods contributes to improved immune function, enhanced digestion, and increased energy levels. Additionally, plant-based diets are generally lower in saturated fat and cholesterol, making them heart-friendly and supportive of cardiovascular health.

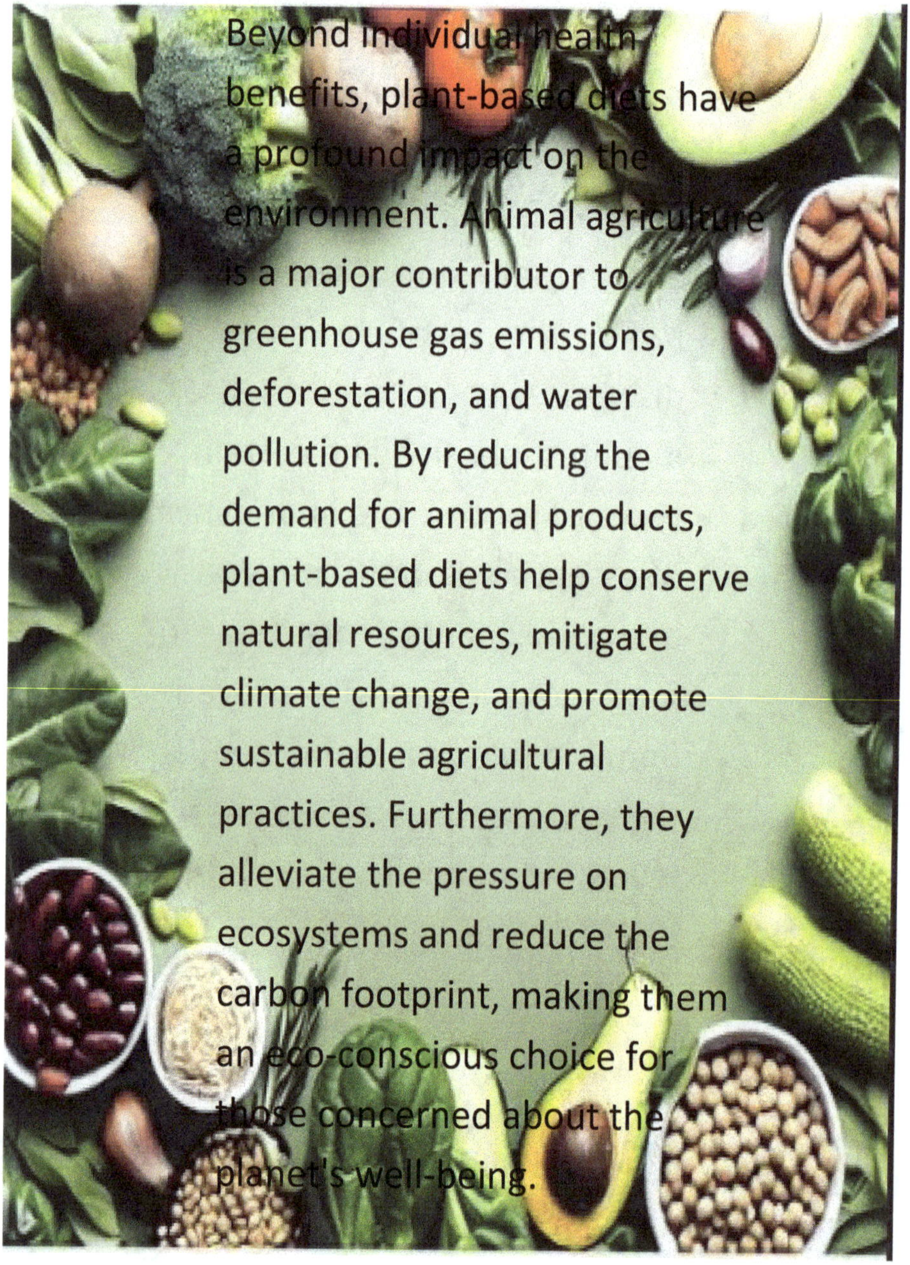

Beyond individual health benefits, plant-based diets have a profound impact on the environment. Animal agriculture is a major contributor to greenhouse gas emissions, deforestation, and water pollution. By reducing the demand for animal products, plant-based diets help conserve natural resources, mitigate climate change, and promote sustainable agricultural practices. Furthermore, they alleviate the pressure on ecosystems and reduce the carbon footprint, making them an eco-conscious choice for those concerned about the planet's well-being.

Ethical considerations also play a significant role in the decision to adopt a plant-based lifestyle. Many people are concerned about the welfare of animals raised for food and the ethics of their treatment in the food industry. Plant-based diets offer an alternative that aligns with principles of compassion and respect for all living beings.

However, embracing a plant-based diet requires careful planning to ensure proper nutrition. While plant-based foods are rich in essential nutrients, some may need to pay attention to certain vitamins and minerals like vitamin B12, iron, calcium, and omega-3 fatty acids. Proper education and dietary guidance are essential to meet individual nutritional needs effectively.

In conclusion, the power of plants in plant-based diets lies in their ability to promote better health, contribute to environmental sustainability, and align with ethical values.

As more people recognize the benefits, it is likely that plant-based diets will continue to play a pivotal role in the future of food choices, offering a path towards a healthier, greener, and more compassionate world

Overcoming Common Myths and Misconceptions of a Plant-Based Diet

In recent years, there has been a surge in interest and adoption of plant-based diets due to their potential health and environmental benefits. However, despite the growing popularity, there are still several myths and misconceptions surrounding this dietary choice.

Addressing and dispelling these misconceptions can help individuals make well-informed decisions and embrace plant-based diets more confidently.

1. Lack of Protein: One of the most prevalent myths is that plant-based diets lack sufficient protein. In reality, there are

plenty of plant-based protein sources, such as legumes, tofu, tempeh, nuts, seeds, and whole grains. With proper planning, individuals can easily meet their protein needs through a well-balanced plant-based diet.

2. Incomplete Nutrition: Some believe that plant-based diets are nutritionally deficient and cannot provide all essential nutrients. However, by incorporating a diverse range of plant foods, such as fruits, vegetables, whole grains, nuts, and seeds, individuals can obtain all the necessary vitamins, minerals, and antioxidants their bodies need.

3. Low Energy Levels: Concerns about reduced energy levels on a plant-based diet are unfounded. In fact, many plant-based foods, like fruits and vegetables, are rich in complex carbohydrates and essential nutrients, contributing to sustained energy levels throughout the day.

4. Iron Deficiency: While it is true that plant-based iron sources may not be as easily absorbed as animal-based ones, pairing iron-rich foods with vitamin C sources enhances iron absorption.

   Foods like beans, lentils, and leafy greens can provide ample iron when consumed strategically.

5. Calcium Intake: The belief that plant-based diets lead to inadequate calcium intake and weak bones is misguided. Many plant-based foods, such as broccoli, kale, almonds, and fortified plant-based milk, are excellent sources of calcium.

6. B12 Deficiency: Vitamin B12 is primarily found in animal products, leading to concerns about deficiencies in plant-based diets. However, fortified plant-based milk, nutritional yeast, and B12

supplements can effectively meet the B12 needs of those following a plant-based lifestyle.

7. Expense: Another myth is that plant-based diets are expensive.

While certain specialty plant-based products can be pricey, a well-planned plant-based diet centered around whole foods can be affordable and budget-friendly.

8. Athlete Performance: Some worry that plant-based diets may compromise athletic performance due to insufficient protein intake. However, numerous successful athletes follow plant-based diets and achieve outstanding results, indicating that it is possible to excel athletically without animal products.

9. Lack of Flavor: Contrary to popular belief, plant-based diets can be incredibly flavorful and

versatile. By experimenting with various herbs, spices, and cooking techniques, individuals can create delicious and satisfying plant-based meals.

10.   Social Challenges: Many people fear that adopting a plant-based diet will isolate them socially. However, plant-based options are increasingly available at restaurants and gatherings, making it

easier for individuals to enjoy plant-based meals with friends and family.

In conclusion, while there are common myths and misconceptions surrounding plant-based diets, it is essential to separate fact from fiction.

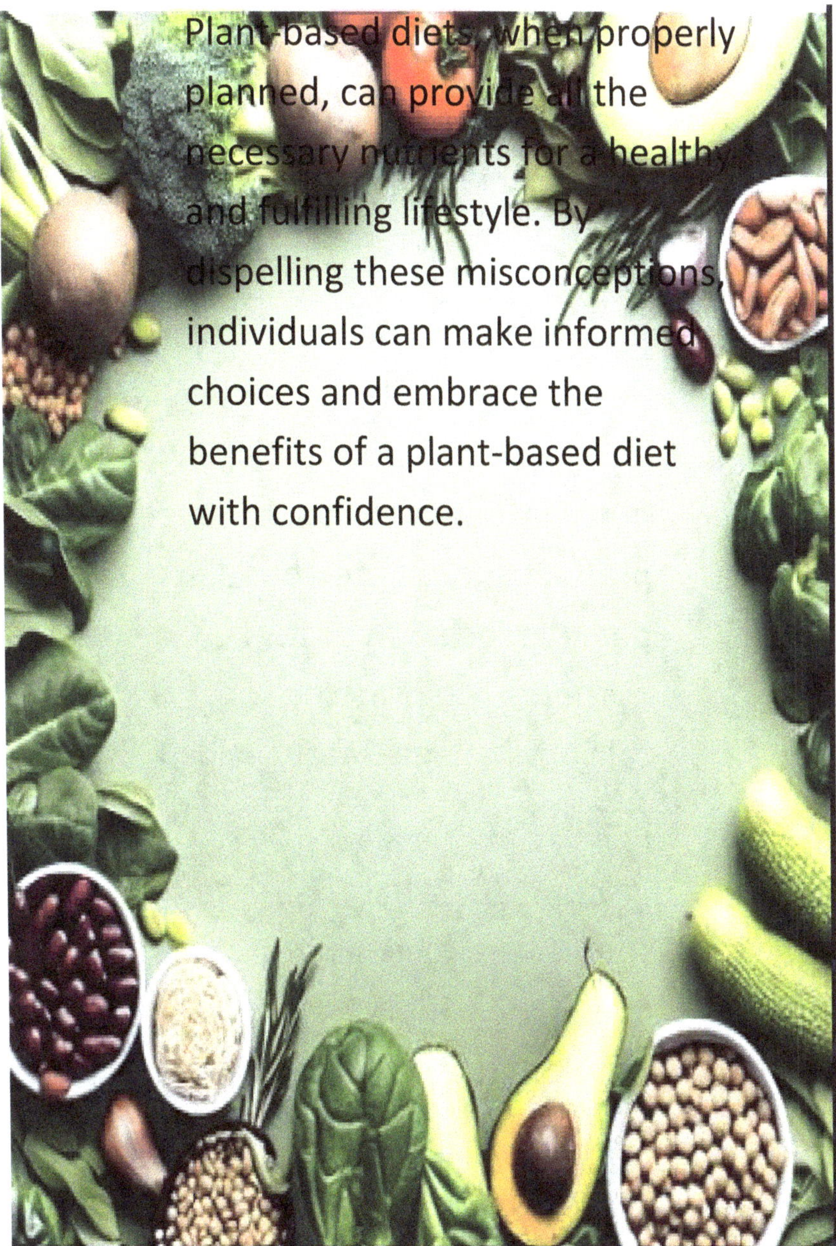

Plant-based diets, when properly planned, can provide all the necessary nutrients for a healthy and fulfilling lifestyle. By dispelling these misconceptions, individuals can make informed choices and embrace the benefits of a plant-based diet with confidence.

Key Nutrients in a Plant-Based Diet (Protein, Iron, Calcium, Omega-3, etc.)

A well-planned plant-based diet can provide all the essential nutrients necessary for maintaining optimal health and well-being. While some may have concerns about meeting nutrient needs without animal products, there are abundant plant-based sources for key nutrients like protein, iron, calcium, omega-3 fatty acids, and more.

1. Protein: Plant-based protein sources are diverse and abundant. Legumes, such as lentils, chickpeas, and black beans, are excellent sources of protein.

Additionally, tofu, tempeh, edamame, nuts, seeds, quinoa, and whole grains like brown rice and oats are rich in protein. By incorporating a variety of these foods, individuals can easily meet their protein requirements.

2. Iron: Plant-based sources of iron include dark leafy greens like spinach and kale, lentils, chickpeas, tofu, pumpkin seeds, and fortified cereals. To enhance iron absorption, it's helpful to consume iron-rich foods alongside vitamin C sources, such as citrus fruits, tomatoes, and bell peppers.

3. Calcium: Building strong bones and teeth is possible on a plant-

based diet with calcium-rich foods like broccoli, kale, collard greens, fortified plant-based milk (soy, almond, or oat milk), and calcium-set tofu. Fortified orange juice and some plant-based yogurts also provide calcium.

4. Omega-3 Fatty Acids: Omega-3 fatty acids are crucial for heart and brain health. Plant-based sources of alpha-linolenic acid (ALA), a type of omega-3, include flaxseeds, chia seeds, walnuts, hemp seeds, and soybeans. The body can convert ALA into other essential omega-3 fatty acids, eicosatetraenoic acid (EPA) and docosahexaenoic acid (DHA), albeit in limited amounts. For

those who may have difficulty converting ALA, algae-based supplements can be a direct source of DHA

5. Vitamin B12: Vitamin B12 is primarily found in animal products, so plant-based individuals need to obtain it from fortified foods like plant-based milk, certain cereals, and nutritional yeast, or through B12 supplements. Ensuring adequate B12 intake is vital for nerve function and red blood cell production.

6. Vitamin D: While sunlight is an excellent source of vitamin D, it may be challenging to get enough in certain regions or during winter. Fortified plant-

based milk and cereals, as well as supplements, can help meet vitamin D needs.

7. Zinc: Plant-based sources of zinc include legumes, nuts, seeds, whole grains, and fortified cereals. Zinc is essential for immune function and various enzymatic processes in the body.

8. Iodine: Seaweed and iodized salt are good sources of iodine for plant-based eaters. Adequate iodine intake supports proper thyroid function and metabolism.

9. Magnesium: Nuts, seeds, legumes, leafy greens, and whole grains are rich in magnesium, which is vital for

muscle and nerve function, as well as bone health.

10. Fiber: Plant-based diets naturally provide abundant dietary fiber, which supports digestive health, lowers cholesterol levels, and helps maintain steady blood sugar levels. Fruits, vegetables, whole grains, legumes, nuts, and seeds are all excellent sources of fiber.

By being mindful of their food choices and incorporating a variety of nutrient-dense plant-based foods, individuals can ensure they meet their key nutrient needs and maintain a balanced and healthy plant-based diet. If needed, consulting

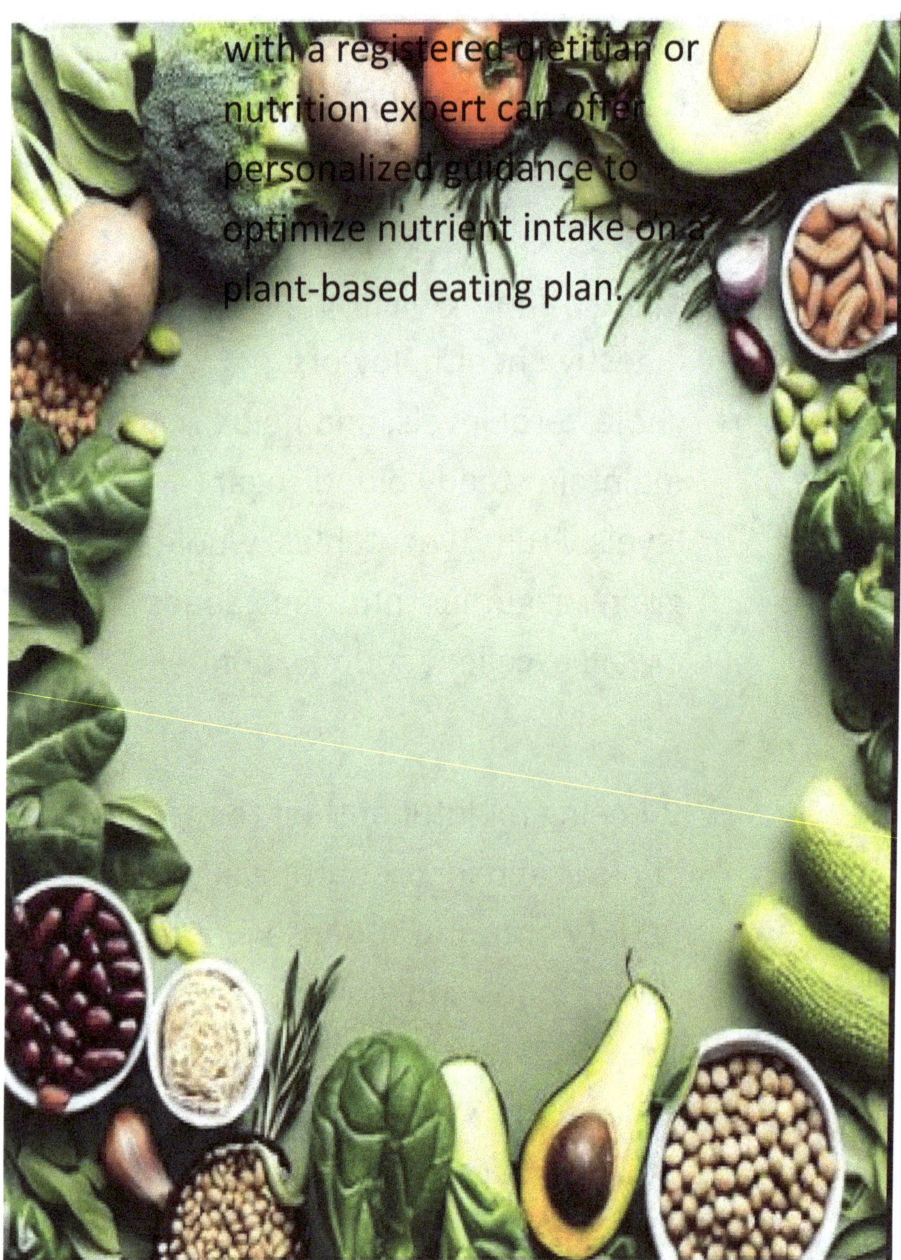

with a registered dietitian or nutrition expert can offer personalized guidance to optimize nutrient intake on a plant-based eating plan.

Transitioning to a Plant-Based Diet - Gradual vs. Immediate Transition: Finding Your Approach

A plant-based diet, which emphasizes whole plant foods while minimizing or eliminating animal products, has gained popularity for its potential health and environmental benefits. Making the switch to a plant-based diet can be a transformative journey, but the approach to this transition can vary from person to person. Two common strategies are gradual transition and immediate adoption. Both approaches have their merits and challenges, and finding the right approach depends on individual preferences, health considerations, and lifestyle factors.

1. Gradual Transition: Gradually transitioning to a plant-based diet involves making incremental changes over time. This approach allows individuals to ease into the new dietary habits, giving their taste buds, digestive system, and mindset time to adjust. Some potential benefits of a gradual transition include:

a. Psychological Adaptation: For individuals accustomed to the flavors and textures of animal-based foods, a gradual shift can be less overwhelming. It allows them to explore new plant-based options at their own pace and develop a deeper appreciation for plant-based dishes.

b. Digestive Adjustment: Changing dietary habits too abruptly can lead to digestive discomfort. Gradual transition gives the gut time to adjust to the increased fiber intake from plant-based foods, reducing the likelihood of bloating or other digestive issues.

c. Sustainable Lifestyle Change: Gradual transitions are more likely to lead to long-term, sustainable lifestyle changes. By adopting one plant-based meal at a time or incorporating "Meatless Mondays," individuals can gradually build confidence and familiarity with plant-based options.

However, a gradual transition can have its challenges. Some individuals may find it challenging to resist the temptation of familiar animal-based foods, leading to slower progress. Additionally, if not carefully planned, a gradual shift may result in nutrient imbalances if certain essential nutrients are not adequately addressed during the process.

2. Immediate Transition: Immediate adoption of a plant-based diet involves a complete shift from animal-based foods to a plant-exclusive diet in one go. This approach requires

commitment and determination but offers its own set of advantages.

a. Rapid Health Benefits: With an immediate transition, individuals can quickly experience health improvements, such as increased energy, weight loss, and improved digestion, especially if they were previously consuming a diet high in processed foods.

b. Ethical and Environmental Impact: For individuals motivated by ethical concerns for animal welfare and environmental sustainability, an immediate transition aligns with their values, as it minimizes direct animal exploitation and reduces their ecological footprint.

c. Clear-Cut Decision: An immediate shift can simplify decision-making, as individuals eliminate all animal products from their diets, avoiding potential confusion about which foods are allowed.

However, the immediate transition can be challenging for some. Sudden dietary changes may lead to cravings for familiar foods, making adherence difficult. Additionally, if not properly planned, individuals may unknowingly miss out on essential nutrients, potentially leading to deficiencies.

Finding Your Approach: The decision between a gradual or immediate transition to a plant-based diet ultimately depends on personal preferences, health considerations, and lifestyle factors. Here are some tips to help individuals determine their best approach:

1. Self-Reflection: Consider personal motivations for transitioning to a plant-based diet. Understanding the reasons behind the change can help guide the decision-making process.

2. Gradual Steps: For those who prefer a gradual transition, start by incorporating more plant-based meals into the weekly

menu and progressively increasing the number of plant-based days.

3. Education and Planning: Regardless of the chosen approach, educating oneself about plant-based nutrition and seeking guidance from registered dietitians or nutrition experts can ensure a well-balanced diet.

4. Flexibility: Be open to experimenting with different foods, recipes, and cooking techniques to discover enjoyable and satisfying plant-based meals.

5. Mindful Eating: Practice mindful eating to develop a deeper connection with food and to be attentive to how various plant-

based foods impact energy levels and overall well-being.

6. Support System: Engage with like-minded individuals or join online communities that share plant-based recipes, tips, and experiences. A support system can provide motivation and encouragement throughout the transition.

In conclusion, transitioning to a plant-based diet can be a rewarding and transformative experience. The choice between a gradual or immediate approach depends on individual preferences and circumstances. Whichever path is chosen, it is essential to approach the transition with patience,

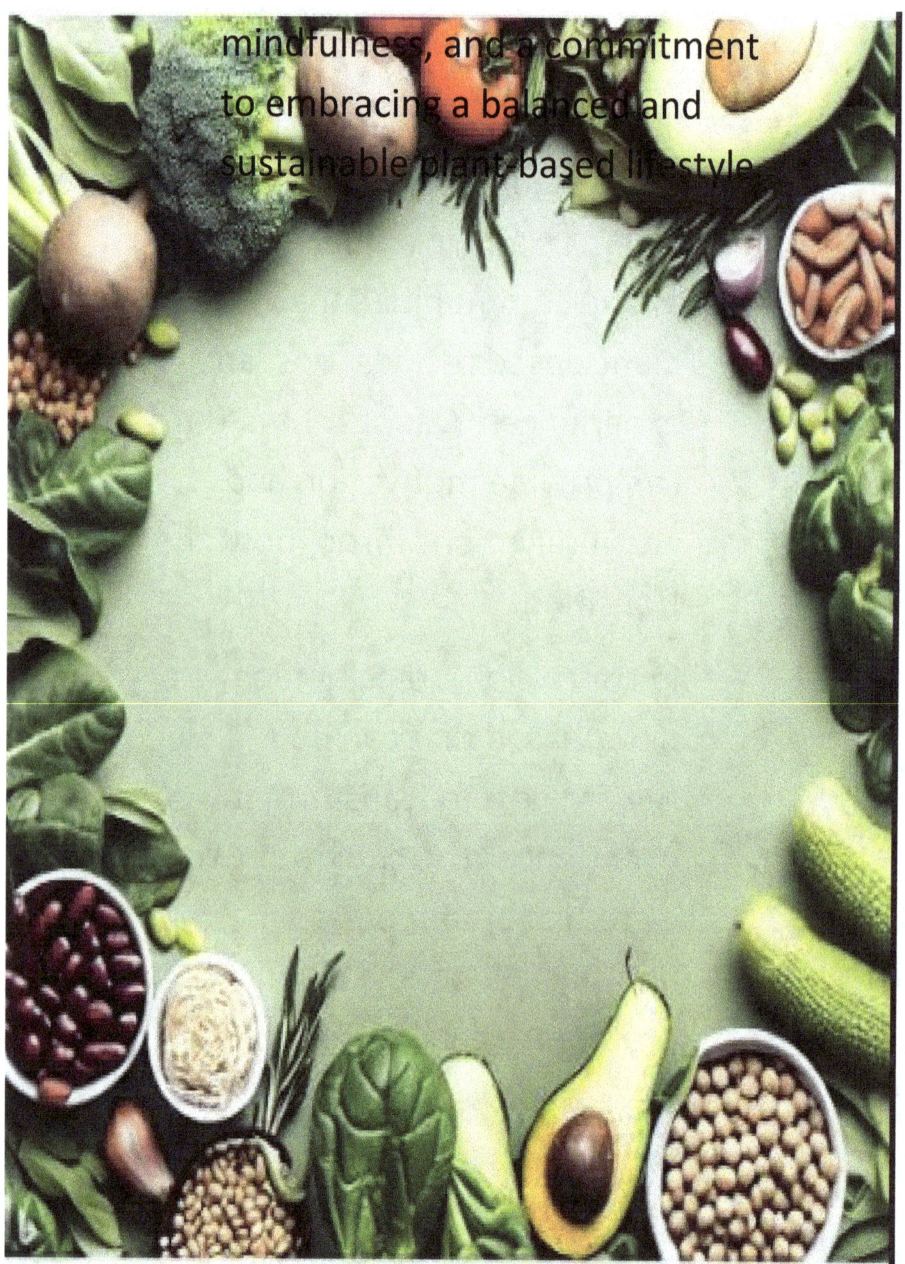
mindfulness, and a commitment
to embracing a balanced and
sustainable plant-based lifestyle

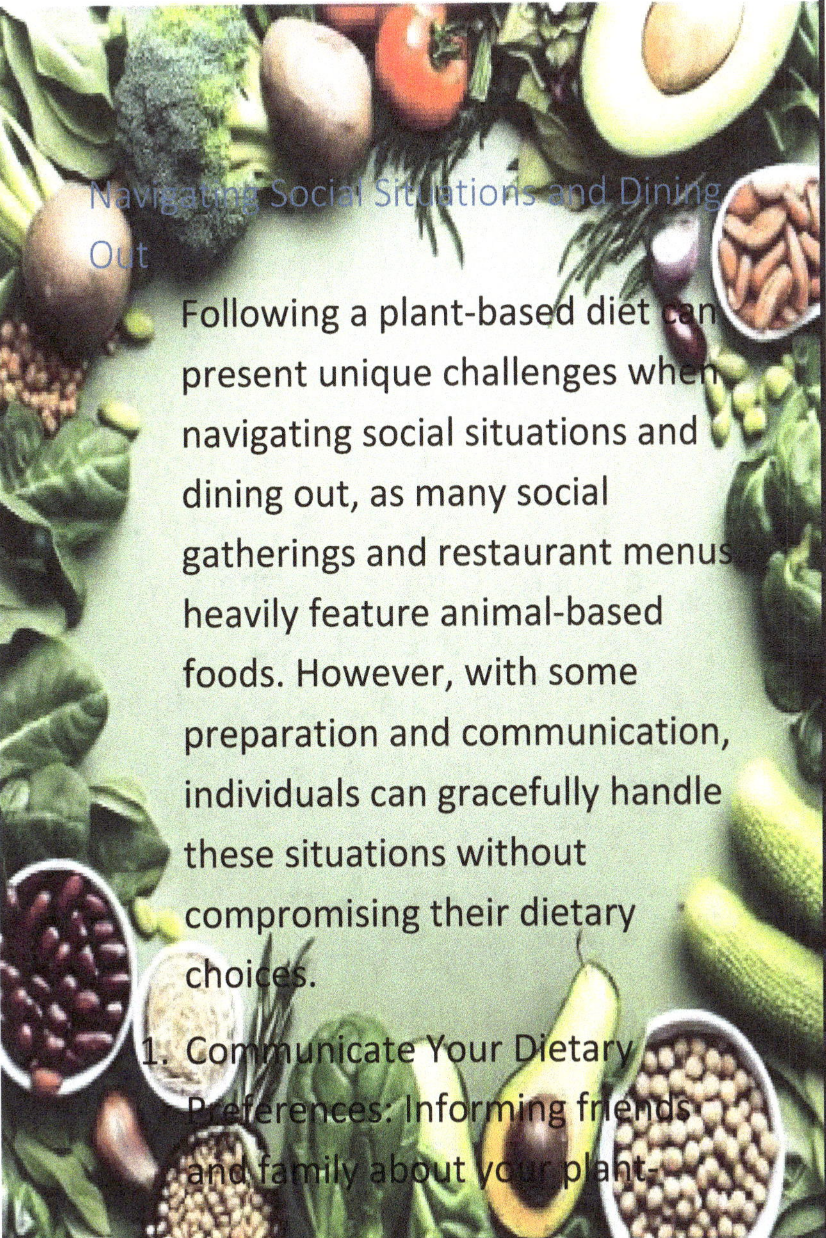

Navigating Social Situations and Dining Out

Following a plant-based diet can present unique challenges when navigating social situations and dining out, as many social gatherings and restaurant menus heavily feature animal-based foods. However, with some preparation and communication, individuals can gracefully handle these situations without compromising their dietary choices.

1. Communicate Your Dietary Preferences: Informing friends and family about your plant-

based lifestyle before social gatherings can be helpful. Sharing your dietary preferences in advance allows hosts to plan meals or choose restaurants that offer plant-based options.

2. Offer to Contribute a Dish: When attending potlucks or gatherings, offer to bring a plant-based dish to share. This ensures there will be at least one dish you can enjoy, and it may also introduce others to delicious plant-based options.

3. Research Restaurants: Before dining out, research restaurants in the area that offer plant-based menus or have customizable options. Many establishments

now cater to dietary preferences and offer a variety of plant-based dishes.

4. Request Modifications: Don't hesitate to ask for modifications to existing menu items to make them plant-based. Many restaurants are accommodating and can substitute animal-based ingredients with plant-based alternatives.

5. Be Polite and Appreciative: If attending an event or restaurant where plant-based options are limited, be gracious and appreciative of any efforts made to accommodate your dietary needs. Thank hosts or restaurant staff for their consideration.

6. Plan Ahead: If unsure about the restaurant's menu options, check their menu online before arriving. This gives you time to plan your order and ask any necessary questions when you arrive.

7. Focus on Plant-Based Staples: When dining out, opt for dishes based on plant-based staples like vegetables, grains, legumes, and tofu. These are more likely to be available and less prone to hidden animal-based ingredients.

8. Communicate with Waitstaff: Clearly communicate your dietary preferences to the waitstaff and inquire about ingredients in dishes. This

ensures there are no surprises and helps the staff understand your dietary needs.

9. Embrace Flexibility: In some situations, it may be challenging to find strictly plant-based options. Be flexible and willing to make compromises, if necessary, while still adhering to your overall dietary principles.

10. Educate and Inspire: Use social situations as an opportunity to educate others about the benefits of a plant-based diet. Share your experiences and favorite plant-based dishes, inspiring others to try plant-based options.

Navigating social situations and dining out on a plant-based diet

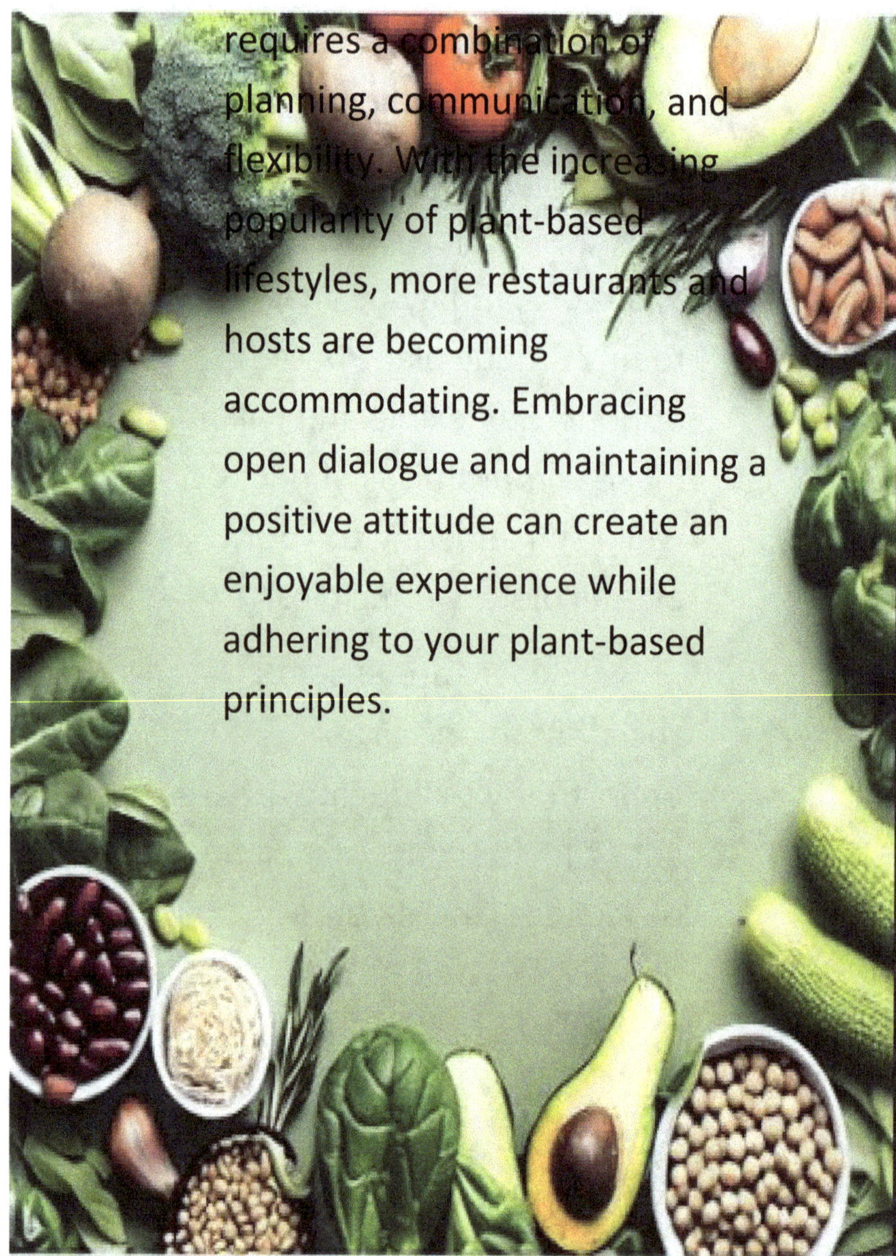

requires a combination of planning, communication, and flexibility. With the increasing popularity of plant-based lifestyles, more restaurants and hosts are becoming accommodating. Embracing open dialogue and maintaining a positive attitude can create an enjoyable experience while adhering to your plant-based principles.

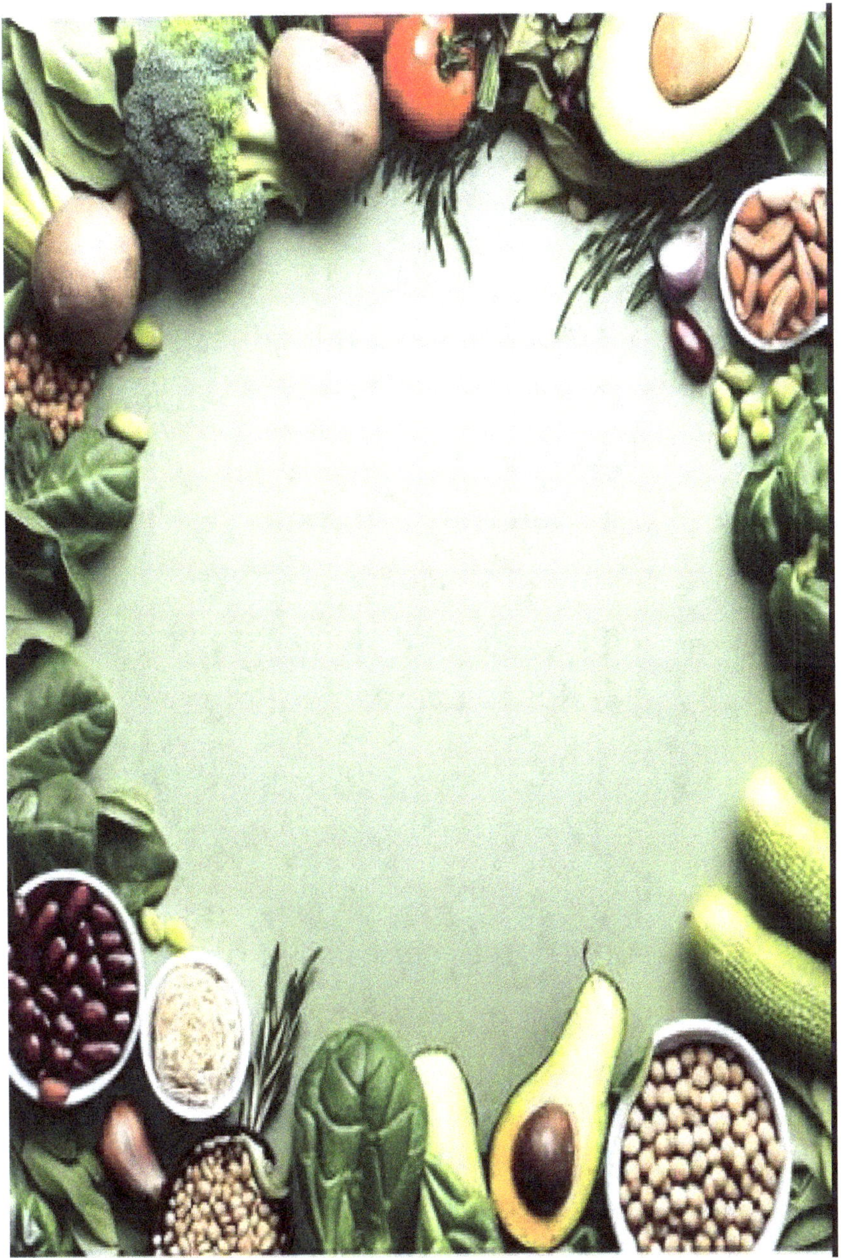

Overcoming Challenges and Obstacles

Transitioning to a plant-based diet can be a transformative and rewarding journey, but it's not without its challenges and obstacles. Overcoming these hurdles requires determination, flexibility, and a positive mindset. Here are some common challenges faced by individuals on a plant-based diet and tips to overcome them:

1. Social Pressure: Social gatherings and events often revolve around food, making it challenging to adhere to a plant-based diet. To overcome this, communicate your dietary choices to friends and

family beforehand, offer to bring a plant-based dish to share, and focus on enjoying the company rather than solely on the food.

2. Limited Dining Options: When dining out, some restaurants may have limited plant-based options. Overcome this challenge by researching and choosing restaurants with plant-based menus or customizable dishes. Don't hesitate to request modifications to make existing menu items plant-based.

3. Nutritional Concerns: Ensuring adequate nutrient intake, especially for nutrients like protein, iron, calcium, and

omega-3 fatty acids, can be a concern.

To overcome this, educate yourself about plant-based nutrition, plan well-balanced meals, and consider consulting a registered dietitian for personalized guidance.

4. Cravings for Familiar Foods: Cravings for familiar animal-based foods may arise, particularly during the transition. Overcome this challenge by exploring new plant-based recipes, finding plant-based alternatives for favorite dishes, and reminding yourself of the ethical and health benefits of your dietary choices.

5. Eating on a Budget: Some may perceive plant-based diets as expensive. To overcome this, focus on budget-friendly plant-based staples like grains, legumes, seasonal produce, and frozen vegetables. Buying in bulk and cooking at home can also save money.

6. Lack of Support: If you lack support from those around you, seek out like-minded communities or online groups to connect with others on similar journeys. Surrounding yourself with support and encouragement can make a significant difference.

By acknowledging and addressing these challenges,

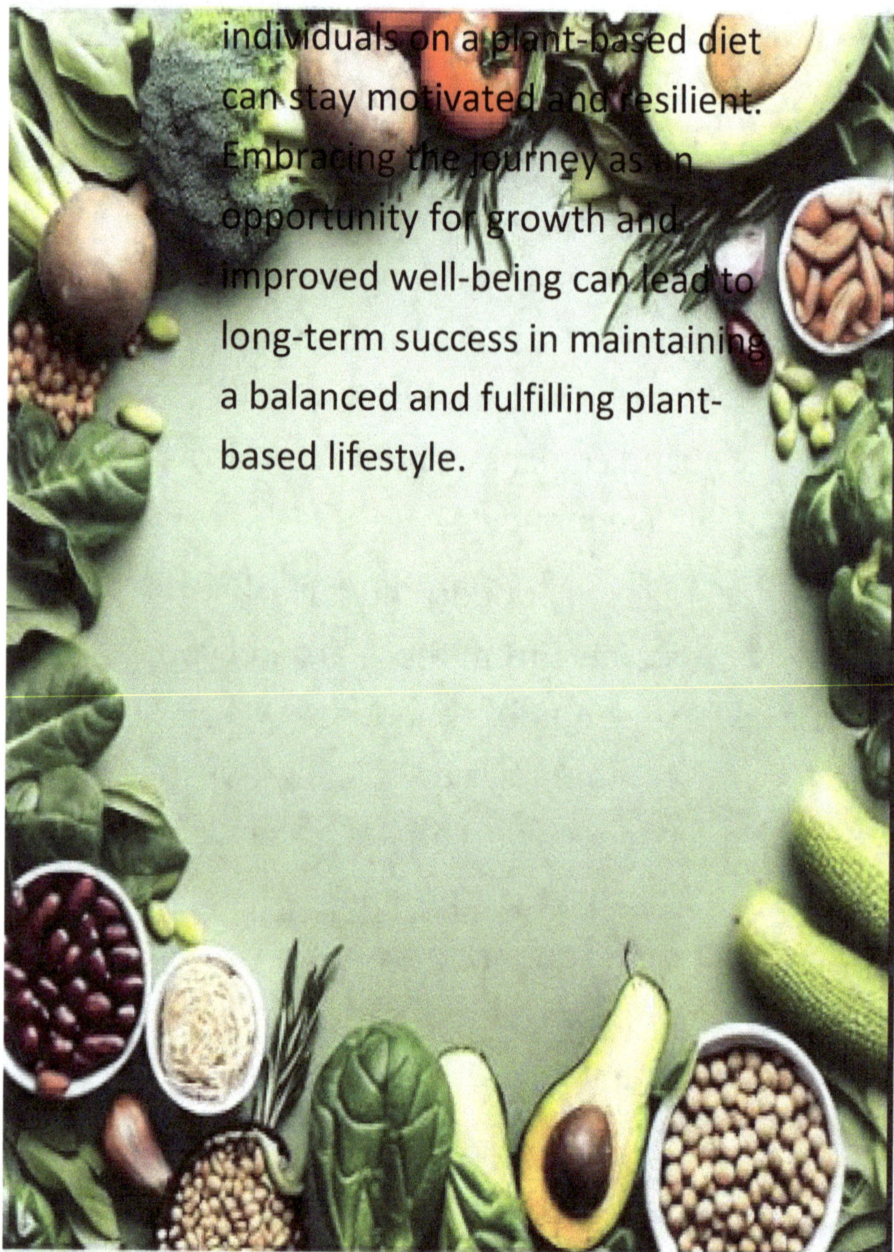

individuals on a plant-based diet
can stay motivated and resilient.
Embracing the journey as an
opportunity for growth and
improved well-being can lead to
long-term success in maintaining
a balanced and fulfilling plant-
based lifestyle.

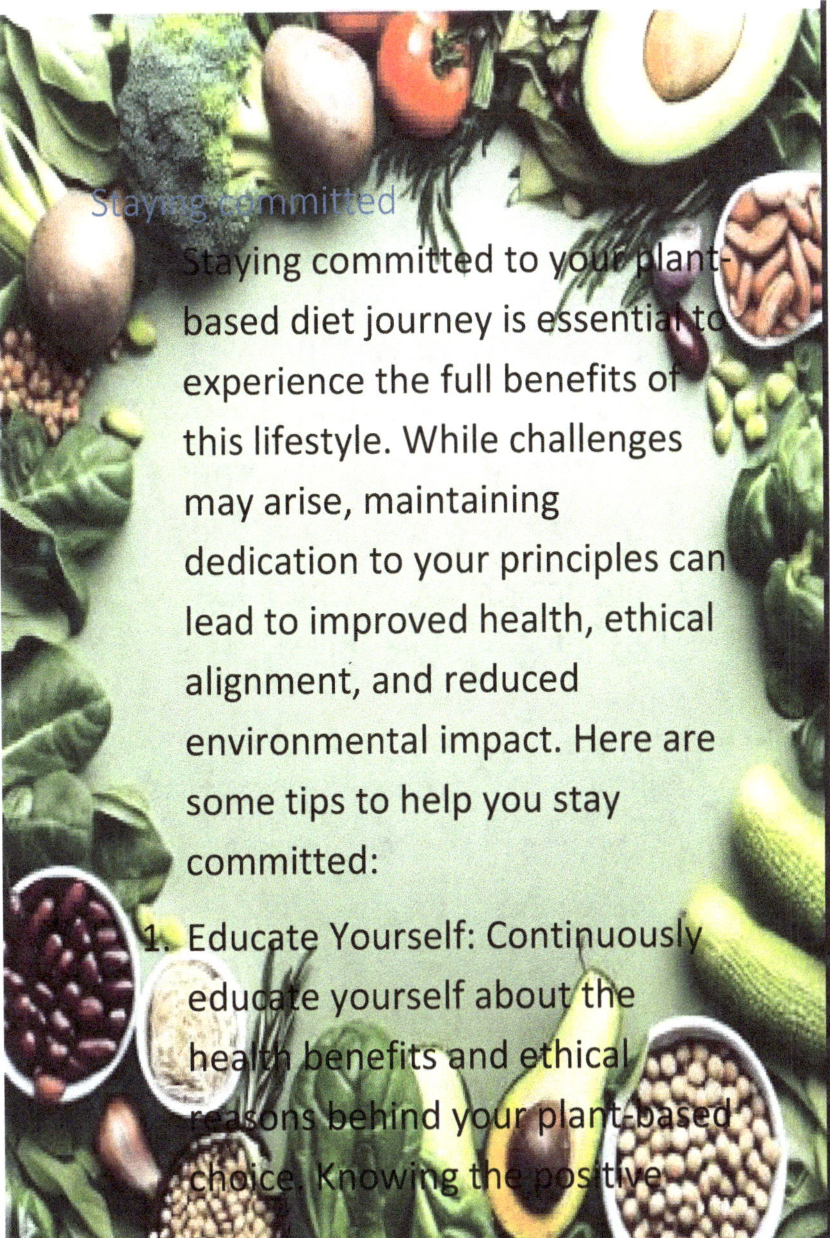

Staying committed

Staying committed to your plant-based diet journey is essential to experience the full benefits of this lifestyle. While challenges may arise, maintaining dedication to your principles can lead to improved health, ethical alignment, and reduced environmental impact. Here are some tips to help you stay committed:

1. Educate Yourself: Continuously educate yourself about the health benefits and ethical reasons behind your plant-based choice. Knowing the positive

impact it has on your well-being and the planet can strengthen your commitment.

2. Set Realistic Goals: Set achievable short-term and long-term goals for your plant-based journey. Celebrate each milestone reached, whether it's trying a new plant-based recipe or successfully navigating a social event with plant-based options.

3. Plan Your Meals: Plan your meals ahead of time to ensure a balanced and satisfying diet. Experiment with new recipes and incorporate a variety of plant-based foods to keep meals enjoyable.

4. Find Support: Surround yourself with a supportive community of like-minded individuals. Join online groups, attend plant-based events, or connect with friends and family who share or respect your dietary choices.

5. Embrace Flexibility: Be flexible and forgiving with yourself. If you have an occasional slip-up, understand that it's part of the learning process. Focus on progress, not perfection.

6. Practice Mindfulness: Be mindful of how your body feels and the positive changes you experience on a plant-based diet. Tune into the benefits you notice, such as increased energy, improved

digestion, or weight management.

7. Seek Inspiration: Follow plant-based influencers, chefs, and experts for inspiration and motivation. Learning from others' experiences can fuel your commitment.

8. Remind Yourself of Your Values: Regularly revisit the reasons why you chose a plant-based lifestyle, whether for health, ethical, or environmental reasons. Keep those values at the forefront of your journey.

9. Avoid Comparison: Everyone's plant-based journey is unique. Avoid comparing yourself to

others and focus on your progress and growth.

10.	Be Patient: Rome wasn't built in a day, and transitioning to a plant-based diet is a process. Be patient with yourself and embrace the journey, knowing that each step forward is a positive change.

By staying committed to your plant-based diet journey, you can make a lasting positive impact on your health, the welfare of animals, and the environment. Embrace the challenges and celebrate the victories, as each moment brings you closer to a fulfilling and compassionate lifestyle.

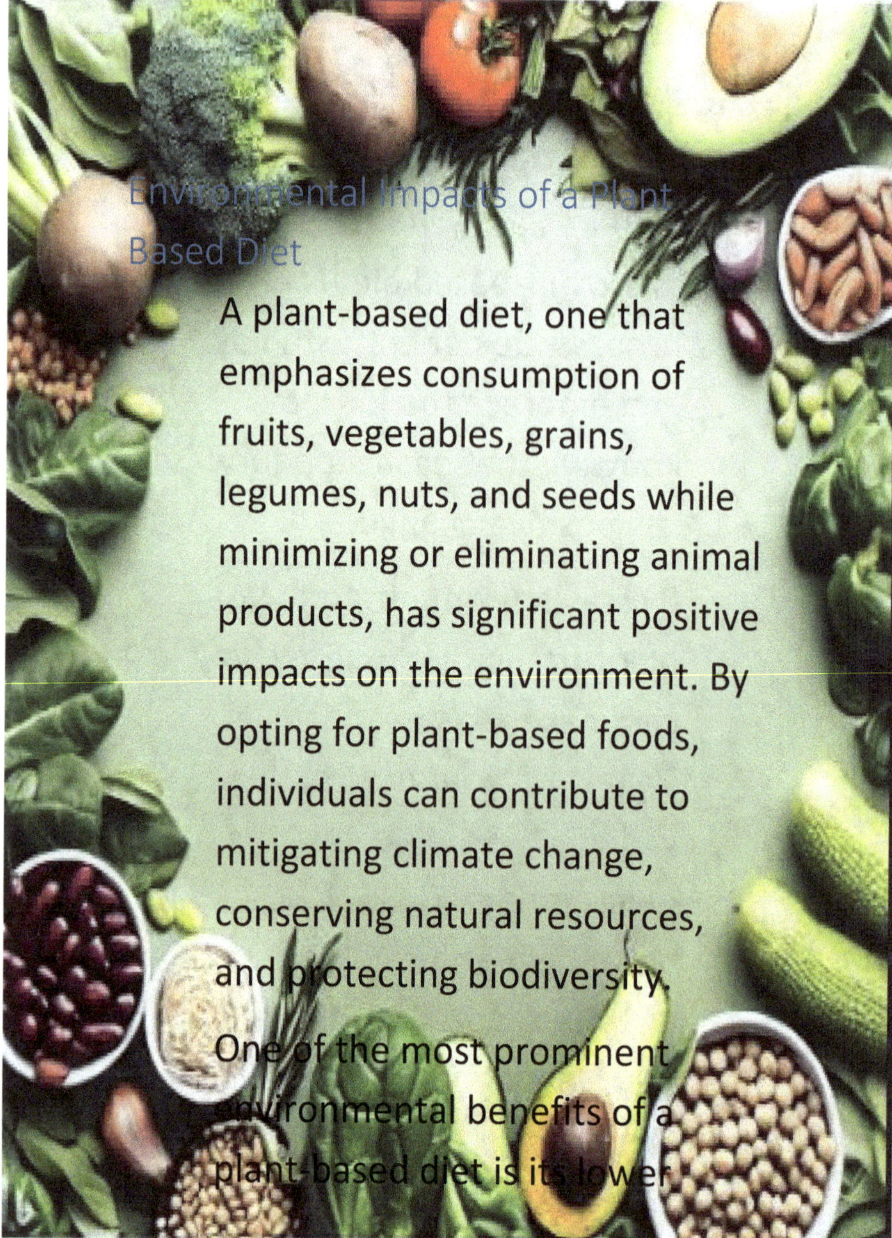

Environmental Impacts of a Plant-Based Diet

A plant-based diet, one that emphasizes consumption of fruits, vegetables, grains, legumes, nuts, and seeds while minimizing or eliminating animal products, has significant positive impacts on the environment. By opting for plant-based foods, individuals can contribute to mitigating climate change, conserving natural resources, and protecting biodiversity.

One of the most prominent environmental benefits of a plant-based diet is its lower carbon footprint. Animal agriculture is a major contributor to greenhouse gas emissions, such as methane and nitrous oxide, which trap heat in the atmosphere and contribute to global

warming. By reducing reliance on livestock farming, a plant-based diet can substantially lower these emissions and help combat climate change.

Additionally, a plant-based diet requires less land, water, and energy compared to animal-based diets. Livestock farming demands vast amounts of land for grazing and feed crops, leading to deforestation and habitat destruction. In contrast, plant-based agriculture is more efficient, requiring less land to produce the same amount of food. Moreover, plant-based diets generally consume less water and energy in the production and processing of food.

Furthermore, a shift to plant-based diets can promote biodiversity conservation. Livestock farming often leads to monoculture practices that result in the loss of diverse ecosystems. Choosing plant-based foods allows for more sustainable agricultural practices that support biodiversity and preserve natural habitats.

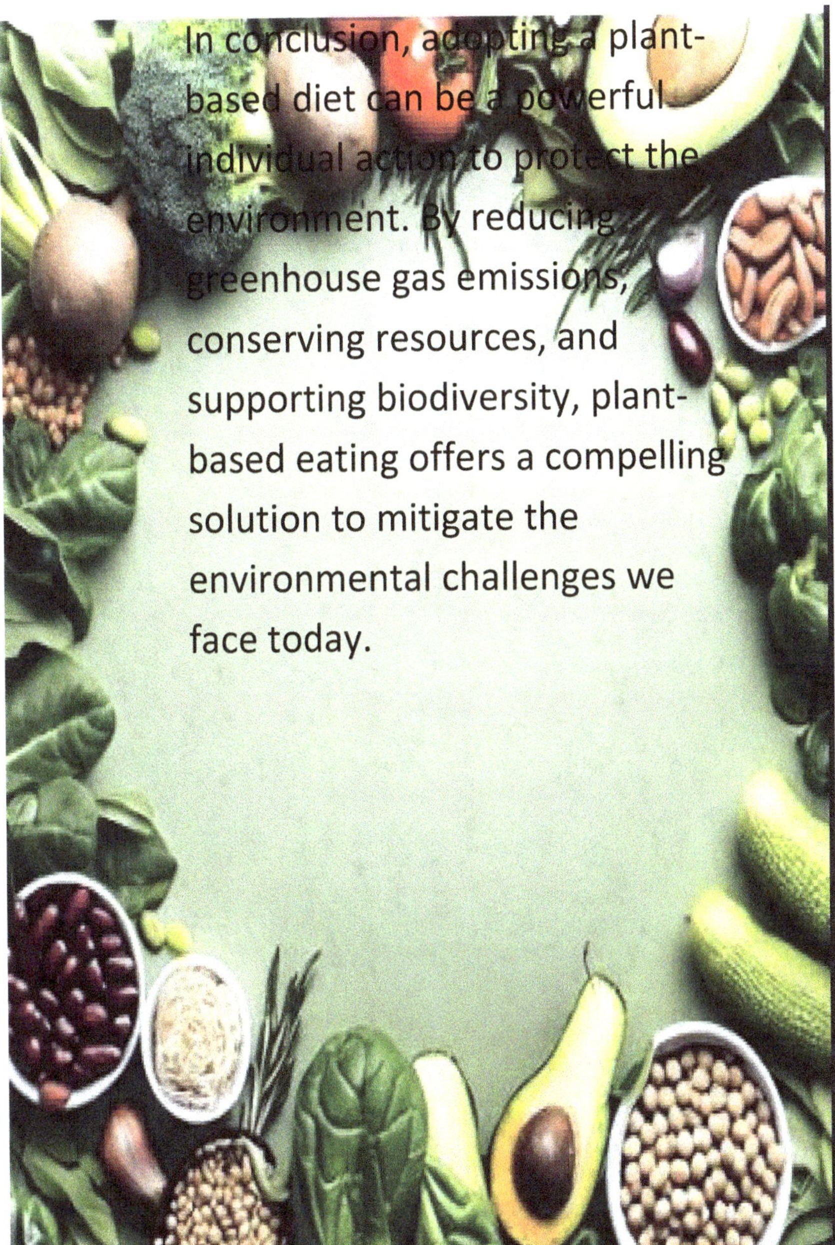

In conclusion, adopting a plant-based diet can be a powerful individual action to protect the environment. By reducing greenhouse gas emissions, conserving resources, and supporting biodiversity, plant-based eating offers a compelling solution to mitigate the environmental challenges we face today.

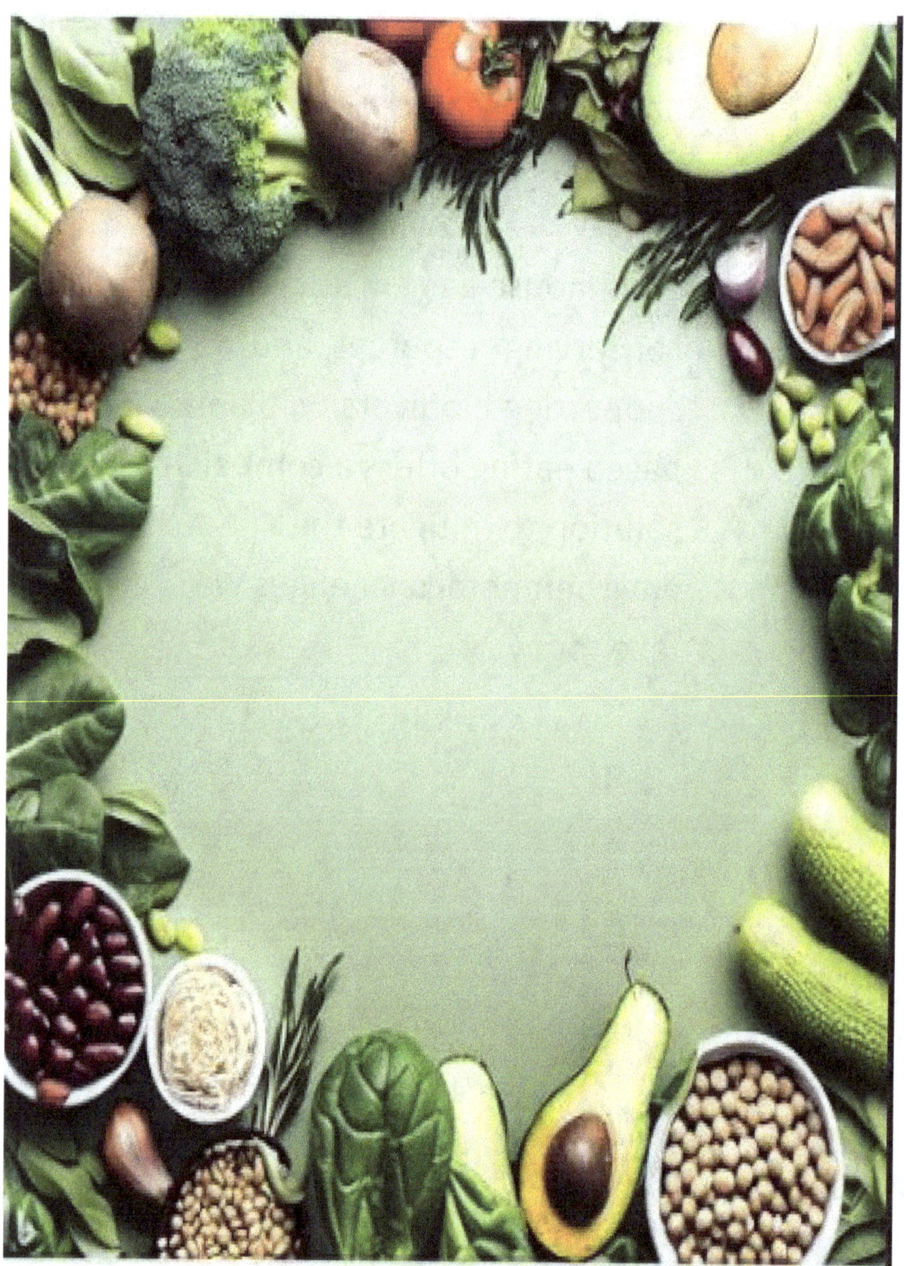

Plant-Based Diet for Older Adults

Plant-based diets have gained significant popularity in recent years due to their potential health benefits, and they can be especially beneficial for older adults. As people age, their nutritional needs change, and adopting a plant-based diet can support overall health and well-being in this population.

Plant-based diets primarily consist of fruits, vegetables, whole grains, legumes, nuts, and seeds, while minimizing or eliminating animal products. For older adults, this type of diet can help reduce the risk of chronic diseases such as heart disease, type 2 diabetes, hypertension and

certain types of cancer. Additionally, plant-based diets are often lower in saturated fats and cholesterol, which can be advantageous for older adults with a higher risk of cardiovascular issues.

One of the key advantages of a plant-based diet for older adults is its potential to manage weight and maintain a healthy body mass index (BMI). Obesity is a common concern in the elderly population and is linked to numerous health complications. By consuming a plant-based diet, older adults can naturally limit calorie intake while still obtaining essential nutrients, thus helping them achieve and sustain a healthy weight.

Moreover, plant-based diets are rich in antioxidants and anti-inflammatory compounds, which can be especially beneficial for older adults as they combat oxidative stress and inflammation associated with aging. These properties can promote healthy aging, reduce the risk of cognitive decline, and improve joint health, contributing to better mobility and quality of life.

Older adults often face challenges related to digestion

and gastrointestinal health. A plant-based diet, particularly when incorporating fiber-rich foods, can aid in regular bowel movements and alleviate constipation issues, a common problem in the elderly.

Plant-based diets also support bone health. Contrary to the misconception that dairy products are the sole source of calcium, plant-based foods like kale, broccoli, almonds, and fortified non-dairy milk contain ample calcium. When combined with vitamin D from sunlight exposure or supplements, plant-based diets can help maintain strong bones and reduce the risk of osteoporosis.

Adopting a plant-based diet can also have a positive impact on mental health and emotional well-being in older adults. Certain nutrients found in plant-based foods, such as omega-3 fatty acids and B vitamins, are associated with improved cognitive function and mood regulation.

Before transitioning to a plant-based diet, older adults should consult with a healthcare professional or registered dietitian to ensure they are meeting their nutritional needs, especially regarding vitamin B12, iron, and other nutrients that may require supplementation in a plant-based diet.

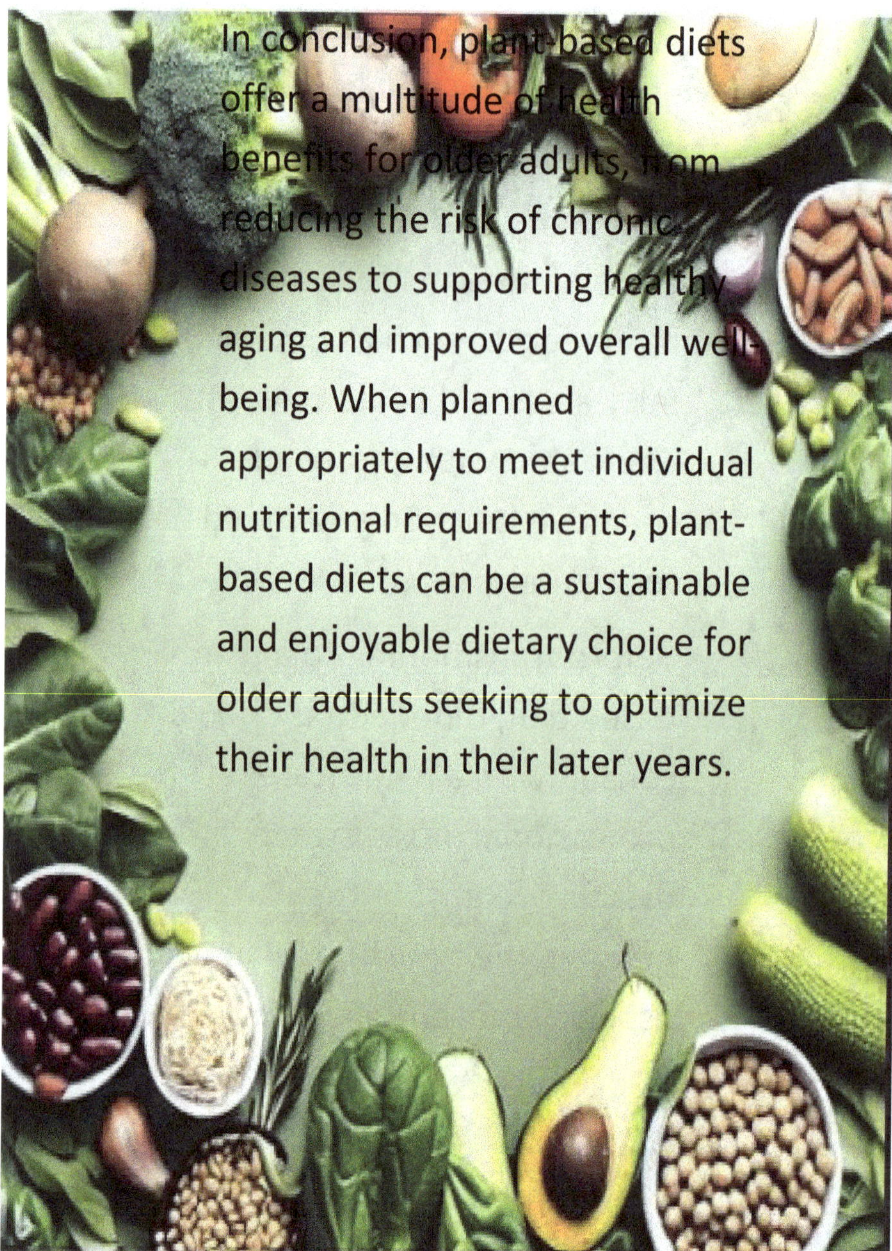

In conclusion, plant-based diets offer a multitude of health benefits for older adults, from reducing the risk of chronic diseases to supporting healthy aging and improved overall well-being. When planned appropriately to meet individual nutritional requirements, plant-based diets can be a sustainable and enjoyable dietary choice for older adults seeking to optimize their health in their later years.

Managing Nutritional Deficiencies

Managing nutritional deficiencies on a plant-based diet requires careful planning and awareness of key nutrients that may be lacking in the absence of animal products. While plant-based diets offer numerous health benefits, such as reduced risk of heart disease, diabetes, and certain cancers, they can also pose challenges in meeting certain nutritional needs. With proper knowledge and attention, it is possible to maintain a well-balanced and nutritionally adequate plant-based diet.

One of the essential nutrients that may require special attention on a plant-based diet is vitamin B12. This

vitamin is primarily found in animal-derived foods, and its deficiency can lead to anemia and nervous system problems. Plant-based individuals can obtain vitamin B12 through fortified foods like plant-based milk, breakfast cereals, or nutritional yeast. Alternatively, vitamin B12 supplements are available in various forms such as tablets, sublingual, or fortified energy bars.

Iron is another crucial nutrient that requires attention on a plant-based diet. While plant sources of iron are abundant, the body may not absorb non-heme iron as efficiently as heme iron from animal products. To enhance iron absorption, it is essential to consume iron-rich foods with vitamin C sources, like citrus fruits or bell peppers. Additionally, soaking, sprouting, or fermenting certain plant foods can help reduce the presence of compounds that inhibit iron absorption.

Calcium is essential for bone health, and while it is abundant in dairy products, plant-based sources can be equally beneficial. Fortified plant-based milk, calcium-set tofu, fortified orange juice, sesame seeds, and leafy greens like kale and broccoli are excellent calcium sources. Vitamin D is also crucial for calcium absorption, and it can be obtained through sunlight exposure or supplements, especially for those living in areas with

 limited sun exposure.

Omega-3 fatty acids, particularly DHA and EPA, are important for brain health and reducing inflammation. While primarily found in fatty fish, plant-based sources like flaxseeds, chia seeds, and walnuts contain alpha-linolenic acid (ALA), a precursor that can be converted to DHA and EPA in the body. However, the conversion efficiency is low, so it is beneficial to consume ALA-rich foods regularly or consider algae-based DHA supplements.

Protein is a critical macronutrient, and plant-based individuals can meet their protein needs by incorporating a variety of plant protein sources. Legumes, tofu,

tempeh, seitan, quinoa, and whole grains are excellent choices. Complementing different plant protein sources can ensure a well-rounded amino acid profile.

Zinc is involved in various enzymatic reactions in the body and is found in plant foods such as legumes, nuts, seeds, and whole grains. However, phytates in these foods can reduce zinc absorption. To enhance absorption, soaking, sprouting, or fermenting plant foods can help reduce phytates' presence.

Iodine is essential for thyroid function and can be obtained through iodized salt or iodine-rich foods like seaweed. However, iodine levels in plant-based diets can

vary, so it is advisable to monitor iodine intake and consider iodine supplements if necessary.

Finally, maintaining a diverse and well-balanced diet is crucial for overall health and preventing nutritional deficiencies on a

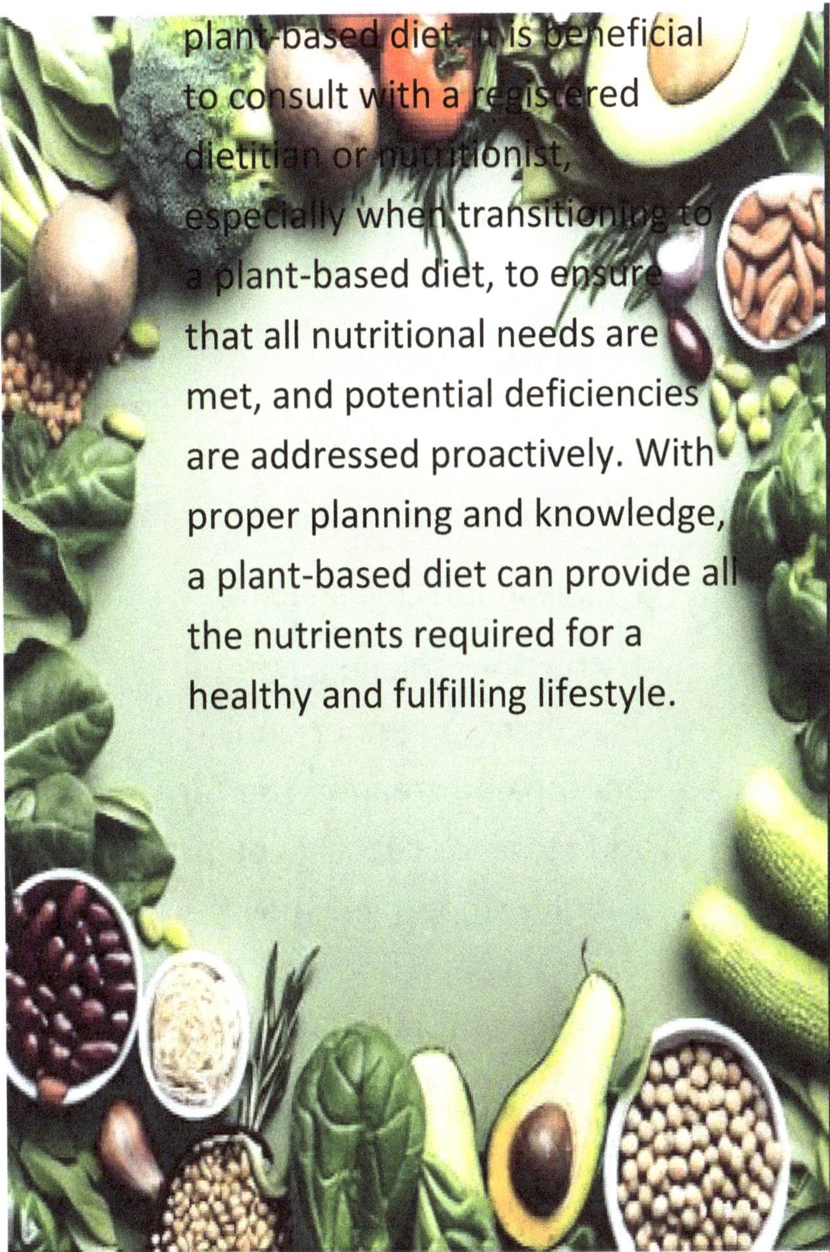

plant-based diet. It is beneficial to consult with a registered dietitian or nutritionist, especially when transitioning to a plant-based diet, to ensure that all nutritional needs are met, and potential deficiencies are addressed proactively. With proper planning and knowledge, a plant-based diet can provide all the nutrients required for a healthy and fulfilling lifestyle.

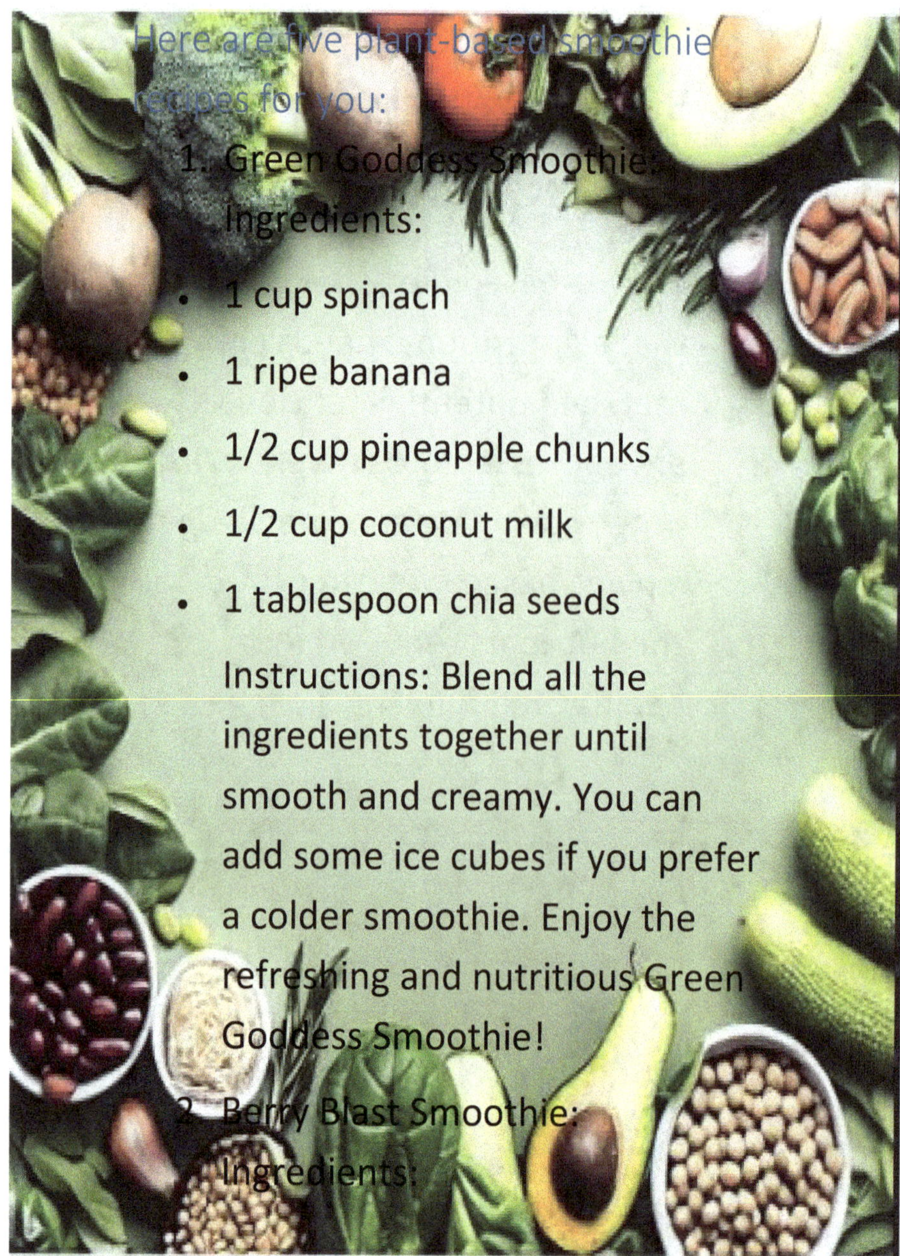

Here are five plant-based smoothie recipes for you:

1. Green Goddess Smoothie:

Ingredients:

- 1 cup spinach

- 1 ripe banana

- 1/2 cup pineapple chunks

- 1/2 cup coconut milk

- 1 tablespoon chia seeds

Instructions: Blend all the ingredients together until smooth and creamy. You can add some ice cubes if you prefer a colder smoothie. Enjoy the refreshing and nutritious Green Goddess Smoothie!

2. Berry Blast Smoothie:

Ingredients:

- 1 cup mixed berries (strawberries, blueberries, raspberries)
- 1/2 cup almond milk
- 1/2 cup plain Greek yogurt (or dairy-free yogurt for a vegan option)
- 1 tablespoon honey or maple syrup (optional, for sweetness)

Instructions: Blend all the ingredients until well combined and creamy. Adjust the sweetness according to your taste preferences. This smoothie is packed with antioxidants from the berries and provides a burst of fruity flavors.

3. Tropical Paradise Smoothie:

Ingredients:

- 1 ripe mango, peeled and diced
- 1/2 cup pineapple chunks
- 1/2 cup coconut water
- 1/2 cup orange juice
- 1/2 cup plain or vanilla plant-based yogurt

Instructions: Blend all the ingredients until smooth and creamy. This tropical delight is a perfect way to start your day or enjoy as a refreshing treat on a sunny afternoon.

4. Chocolate Peanut Butter Protein Smoothie: Ingredients:

- 1 ripe banana
- 2 tablespoons peanut butter
- 1 cup almond milk

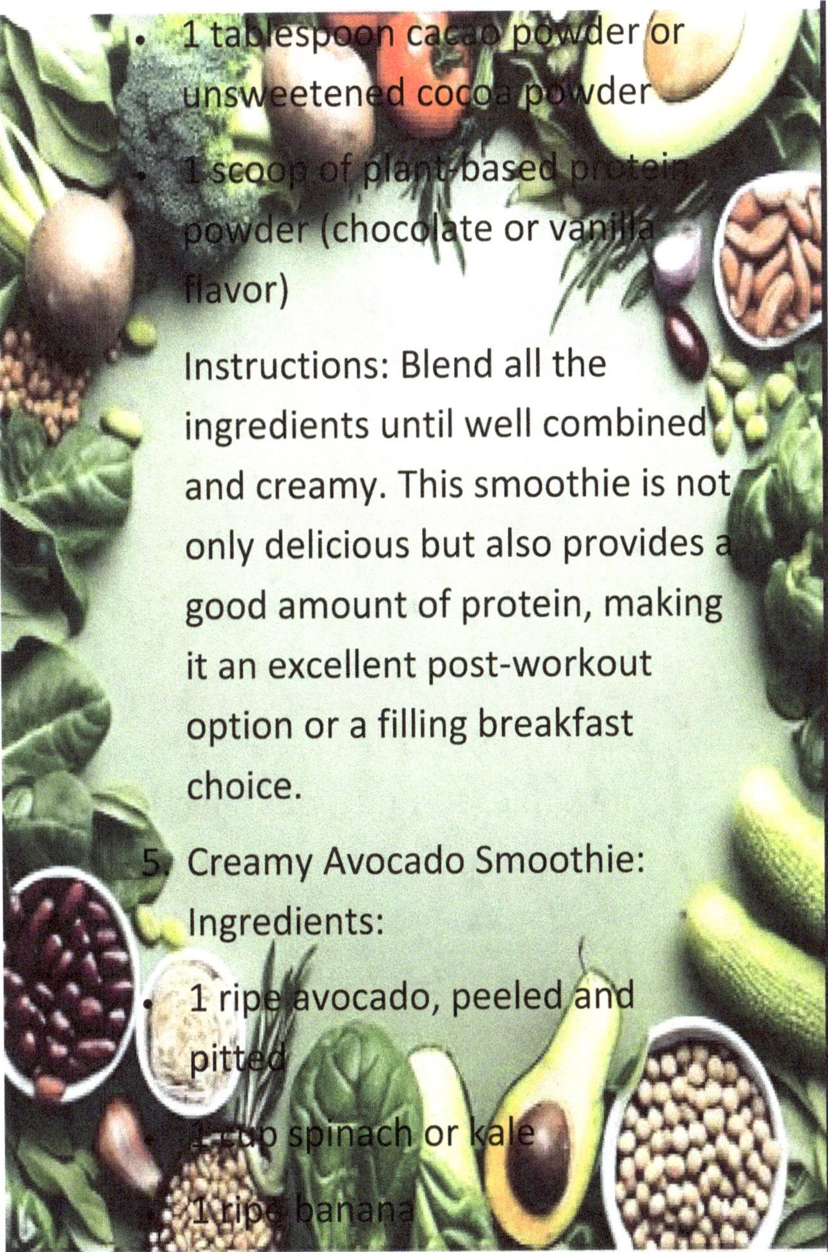

- 1 tablespoon cacao powder or unsweetened cocoa powder
- 1 scoop of plant-based protein powder (chocolate or vanilla flavor)

Instructions: Blend all the ingredients until well combined and creamy. This smoothie is not only delicious but also provides a good amount of protein, making it an excellent post-workout option or a filling breakfast choice.

5. Creamy Avocado Smoothie:

Ingredients:

- 1 ripe avocado, peeled and pitted
- 1 cup spinach or kale
- 1 ripe banana

- 1 cup almond milk
- 1 tablespoon honey or maple syrup (optional)

Instructions: Blend all the ingredients until smooth and creamy. The avocado adds a creamy texture and healthy fats to the smoothie, while the greens and banana provide essential nutrients. Customize the sweetness as desired.

Enjoy these plant-based smoothies as nutritious snacks or meal replacements, and feel free to modify the ingredients to suit your taste preferences!

Here are some meal plans and grocery lists for a plant-based diet. This diet emphasizes whole, plant-based foods such as fruits, vegetables, grains, legumes, nuts, and seeds while avoiding animal products like meat, dairy, and eggs.

Meal Plan #1:

Day 1:

- Breakfast: Smoothie with spinach, banana, almond milk, and chia seeds

- Lunch: Quinoa salad with mixed vegetables and a lemon-tahini dressing

- Snack: Apple slices with almond butter

- Dinner: Lentil and vegetable curry with brown rice

Day 2:

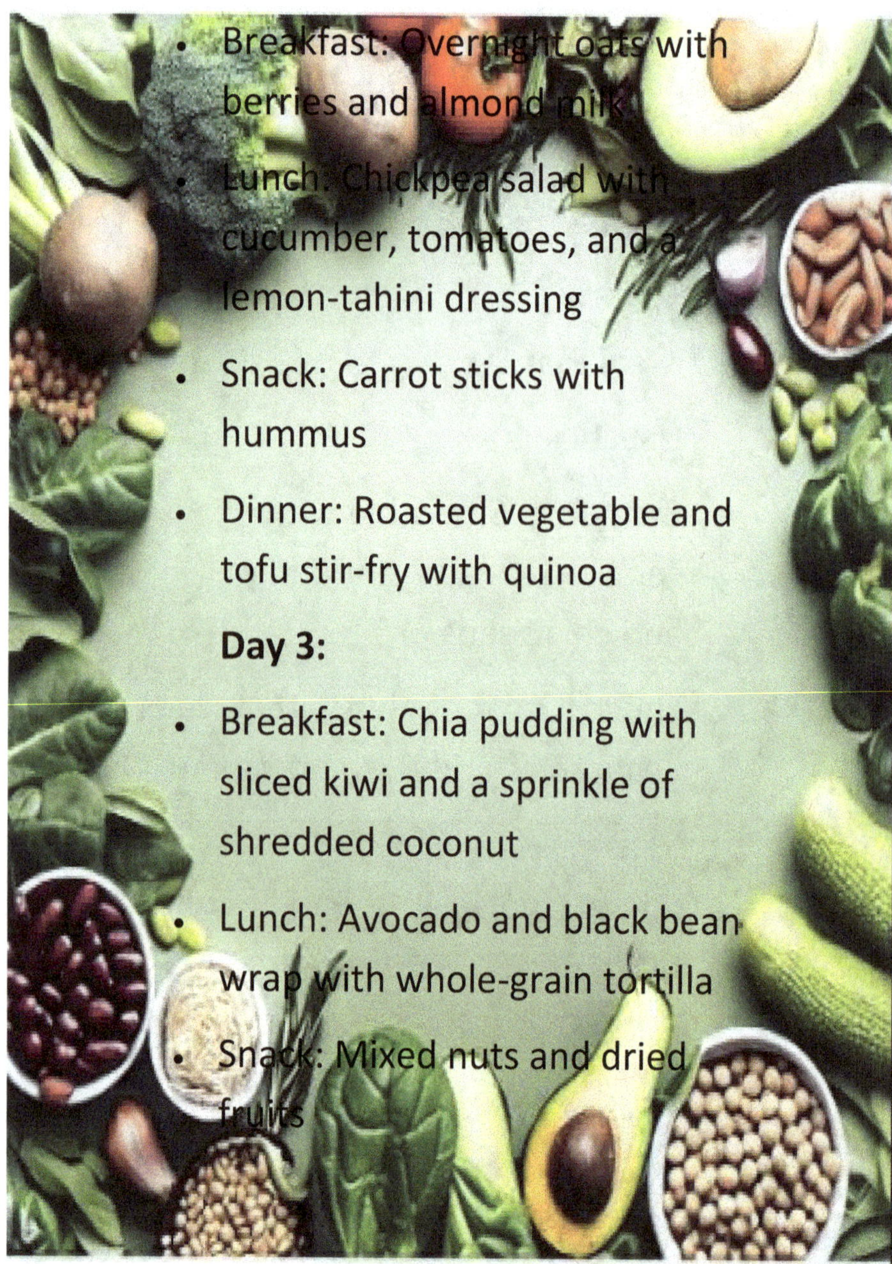

- Breakfast: Overnight oats with berries and almond milk
- Lunch: Chickpea salad with cucumber, tomatoes, and a lemon-tahini dressing
- Snack: Carrot sticks with hummus
- Dinner: Roasted vegetable and tofu stir-fry with quinoa

Day 3:

- Breakfast: Chia pudding with sliced kiwi and a sprinkle of shredded coconut
- Lunch: Avocado and black bean wrap with whole-grain tortilla
- Snack: Mixed nuts and dried fruits

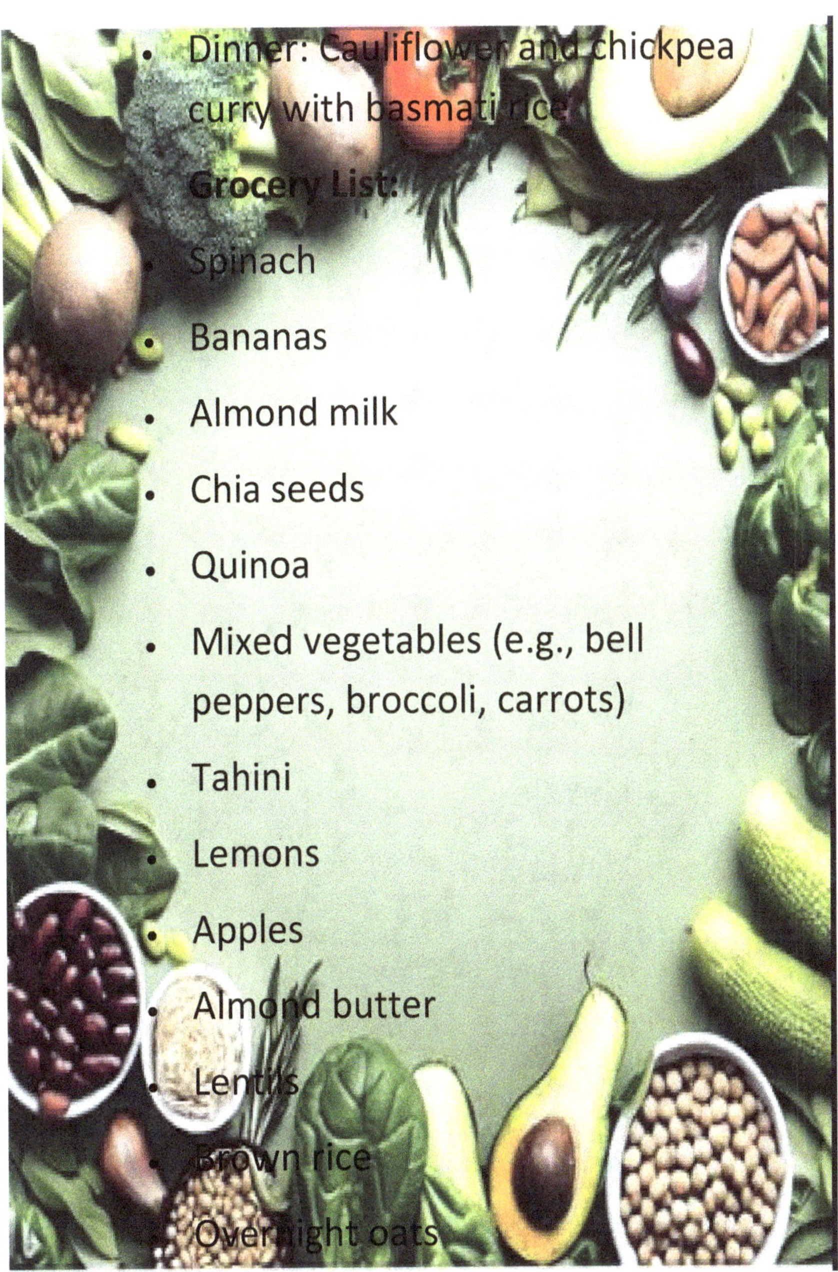

- Dinner: Cauliflower and chickpea curry with basmati rice

Grocery List:

- Spinach

- Bananas

- Almond milk

- Chia seeds

- Quinoa

- Mixed vegetables (e.g., bell peppers, broccoli, carrots)

- Tahini

- Lemons

- Apples

- Almond butter

- Lentils

- Brown rice

- Overnight oats

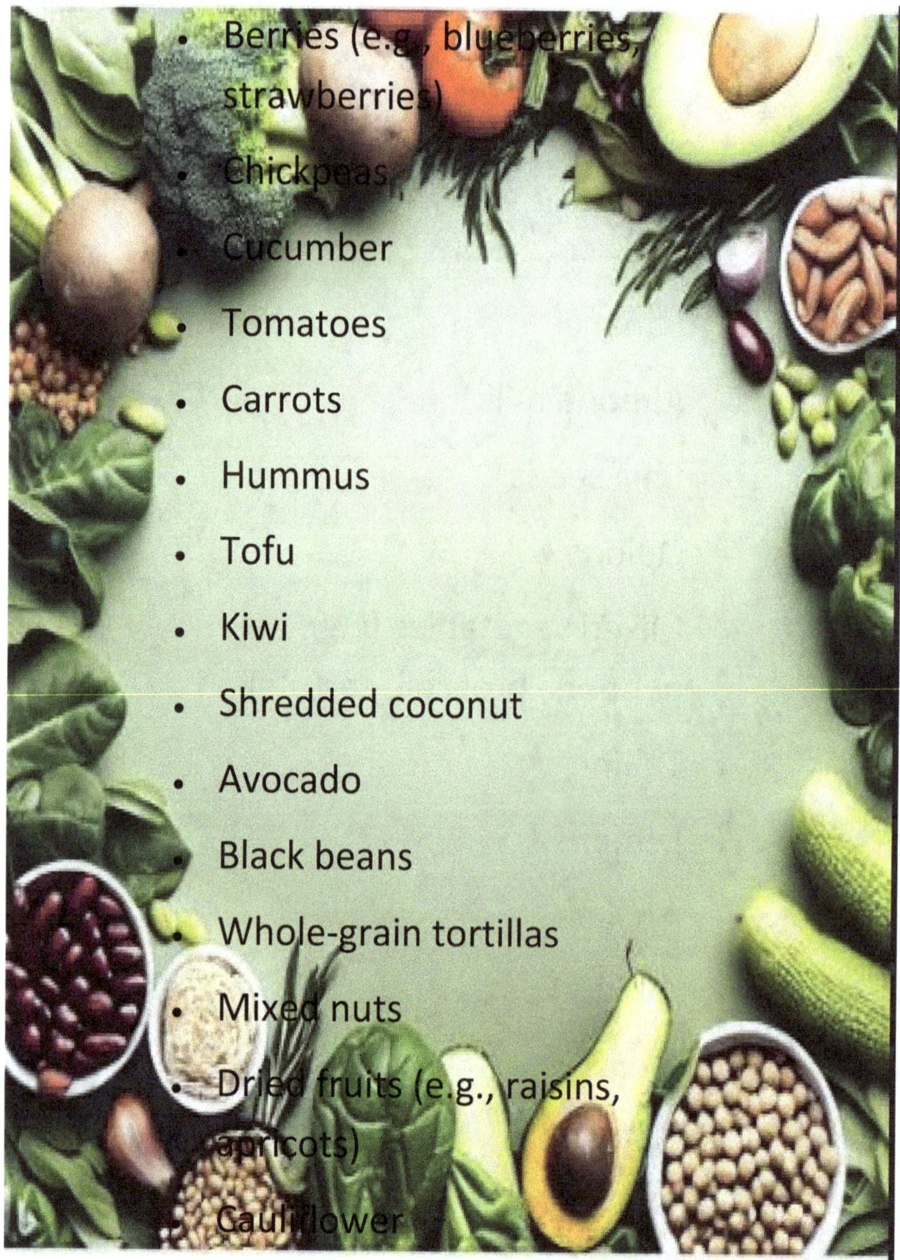

- Berries (e.g., blueberries, strawberries)
- Chickpeas
- Cucumber
- Tomatoes
- Carrots
- Hummus
- Tofu
- Kiwi
- Shredded coconut
- Avocado
- Black beans
- Whole-grain tortillas
- Mixed nuts
- Dried fruits (e.g., raisins, apricots)
- Cauliflower

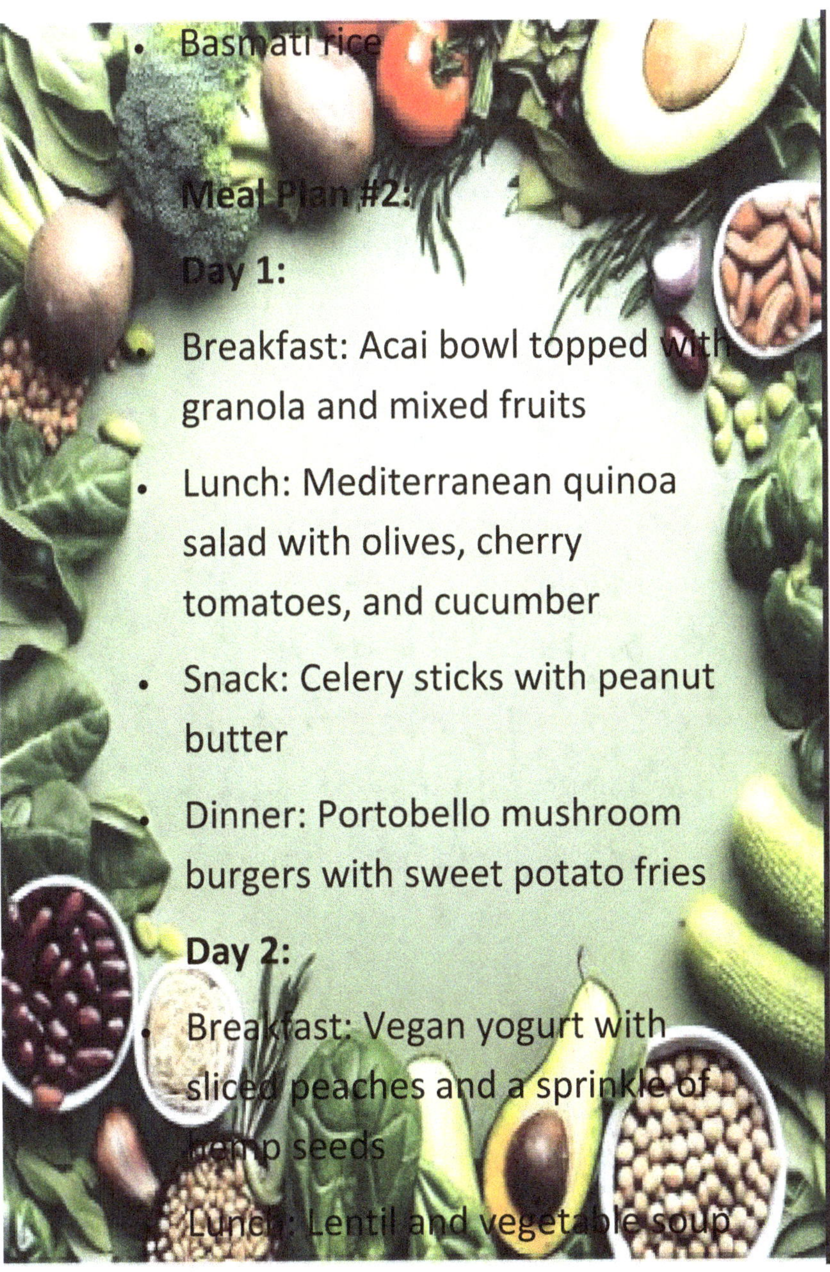

- Basmati rice

Meal Plan #2:

Day 1:

- Breakfast: Acai bowl topped with granola and mixed fruits

- Lunch: Mediterranean quinoa salad with olives, cherry tomatoes, and cucumber

- Snack: Celery sticks with peanut butter

- Dinner: Portobello mushroom burgers with sweet potato fries

Day 2:

- Breakfast: Vegan yogurt with sliced peaches and a sprinkle of hemp seeds

- Lunch: Lentil and vegetable soup

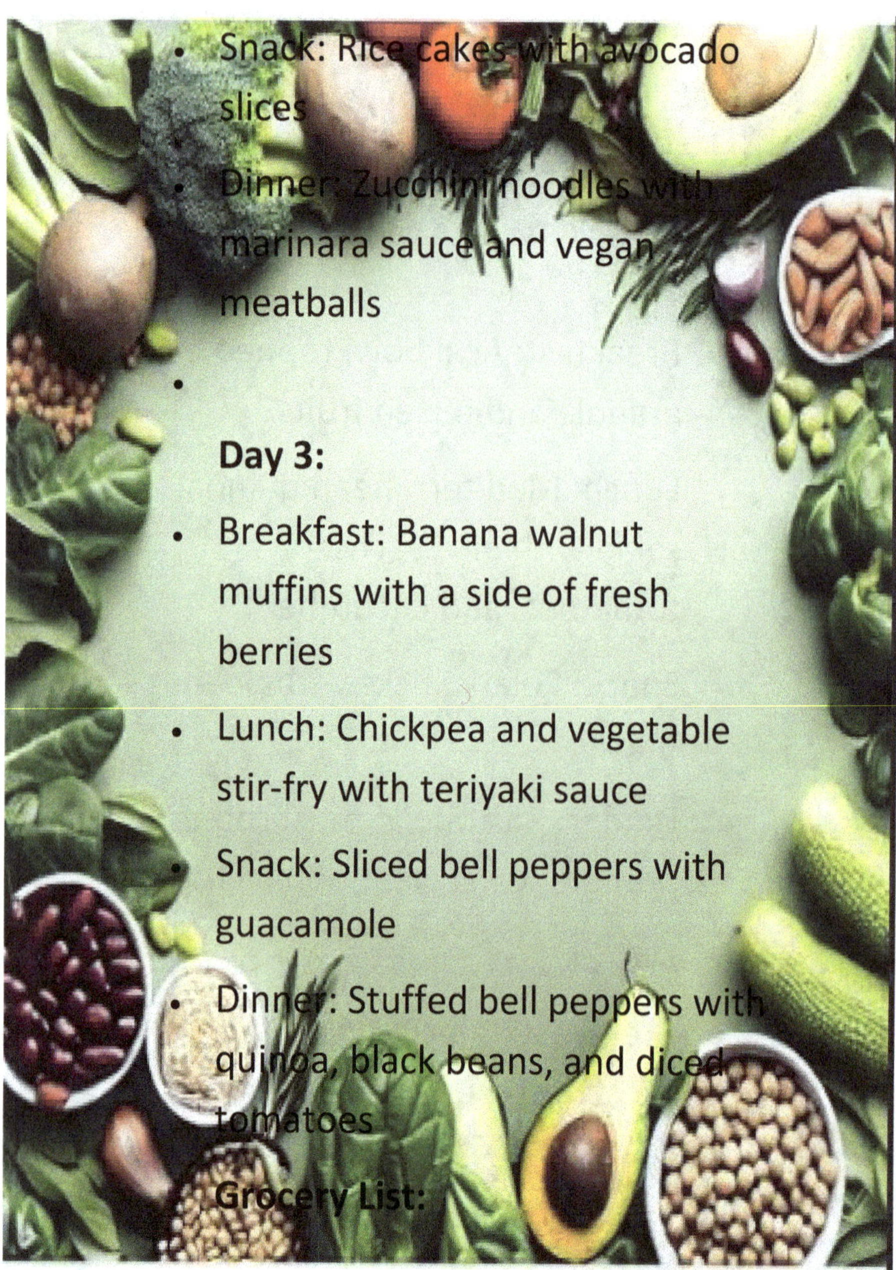

- Snack: Rice cakes with avocado slices
- Dinner: Zucchini noodles with marinara sauce and vegan meatballs

-

Day 3:

- Breakfast: Banana walnut muffins with a side of fresh berries

- Lunch: Chickpea and vegetable stir-fry with teriyaki sauce

- Snack: Sliced bell peppers with guacamole

- Dinner: Stuffed bell peppers with quinoa, black beans, and diced tomatoes

Grocery List:

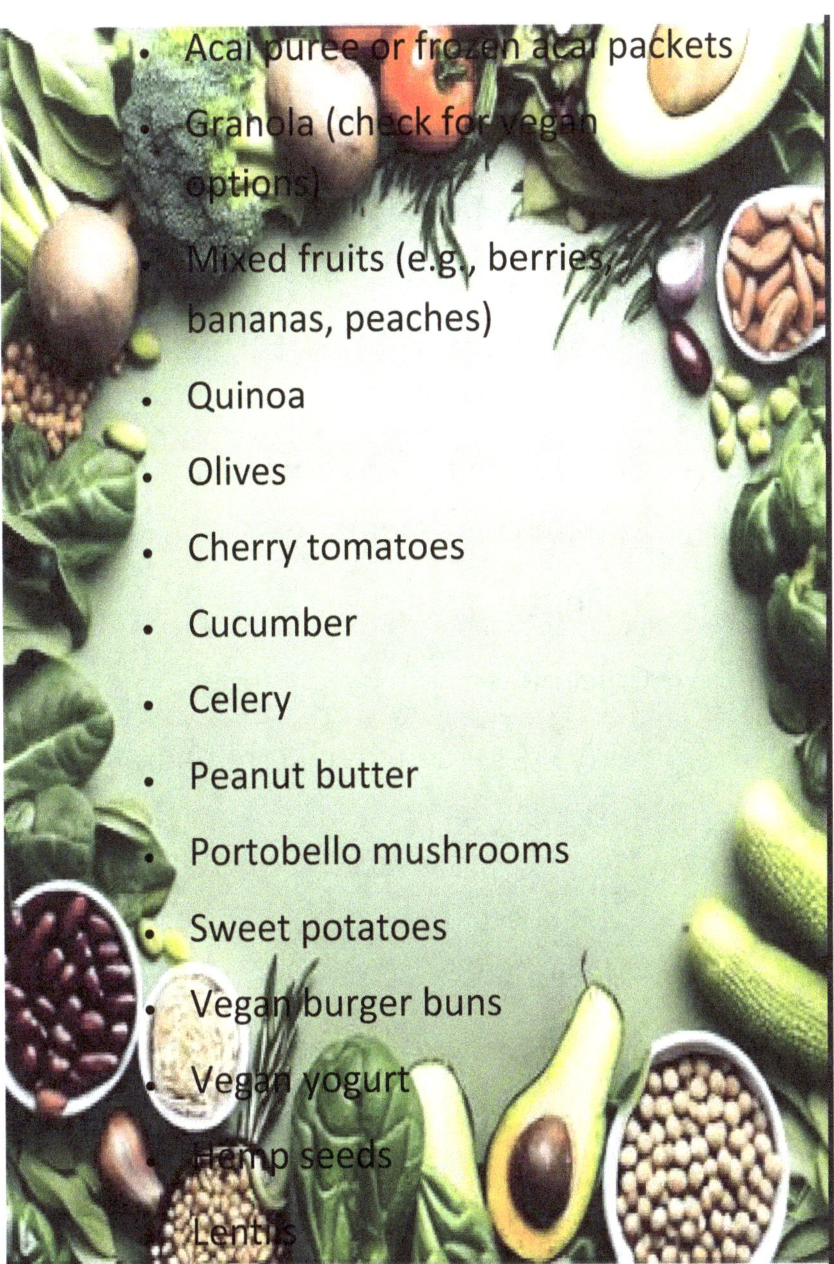

- Acai puree or frozen acai packets
- Granola (check for vegan options)
- Mixed fruits (e.g., berries, bananas, peaches)
- Quinoa
- Olives
- Cherry tomatoes
- Cucumber
- Celery
- Peanut butter
- Portobello mushrooms
- Sweet potatoes
- Vegan burger buns
- Vegan yogurt
- Hemp seeds
- Lentils

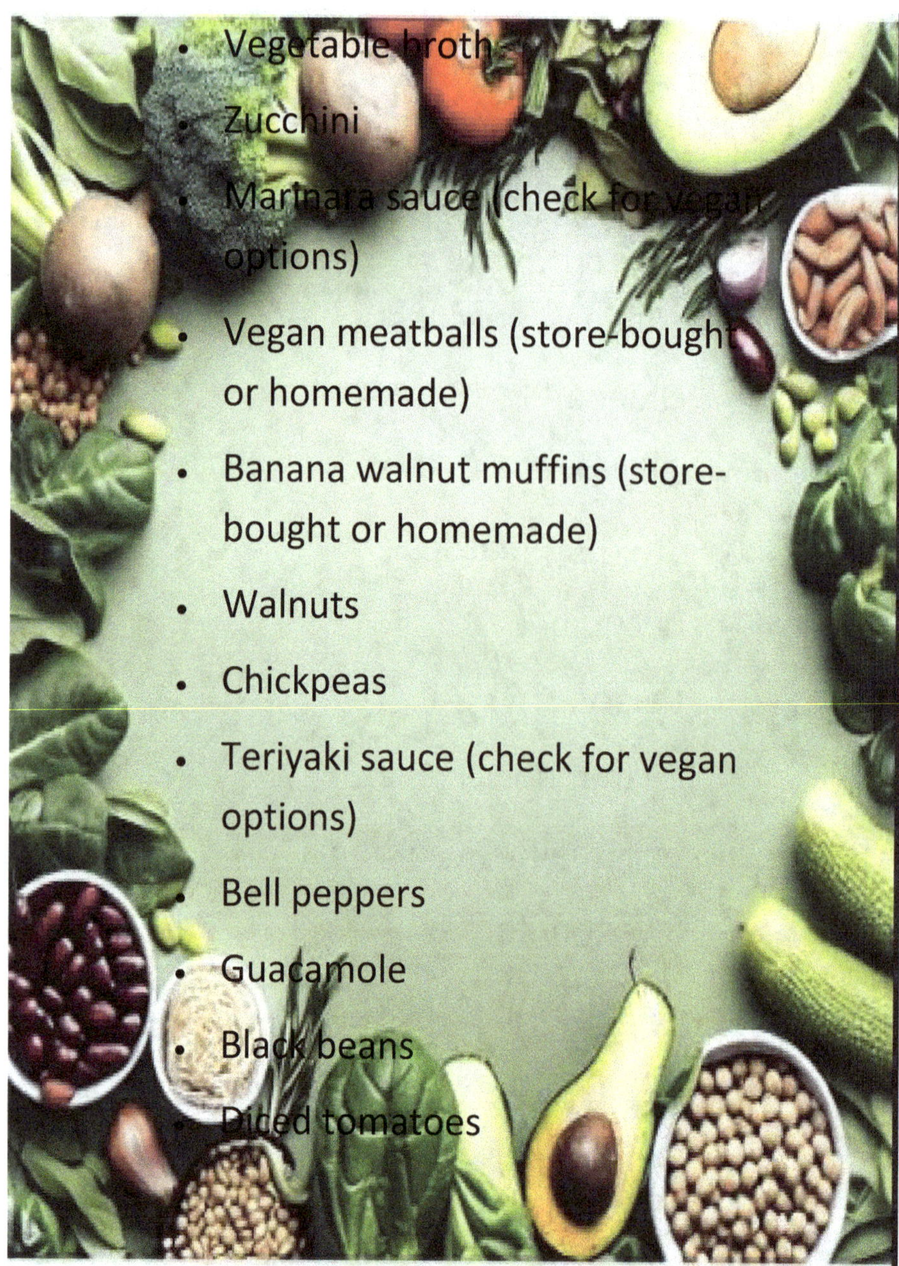

- Vegetable broth
- Zucchini
- Marinara sauce (check for vegan options)
- Vegan meatballs (store-bought or homemade)
- Banana walnut muffins (store-bought or homemade)
- Walnuts
- Chickpeas
- Teriyaki sauce (check for vegan options)
- Bell peppers
- Guacamole
- Black beans
- Diced tomatoes

These meal plans and grocery lists should provide you with a good variety of plant-based meals.

Want More? Here are even more sample meal plans and corresponding grocery lists for a plant-based diet for a week. Please note that these are general suggestions, and you can adjust them based on your preferences and nutritional needs.

Meal Plan #1:

Day 1:

Breakfast: Vegan smoothie (spinach, banana, almond milk, chia seeds)

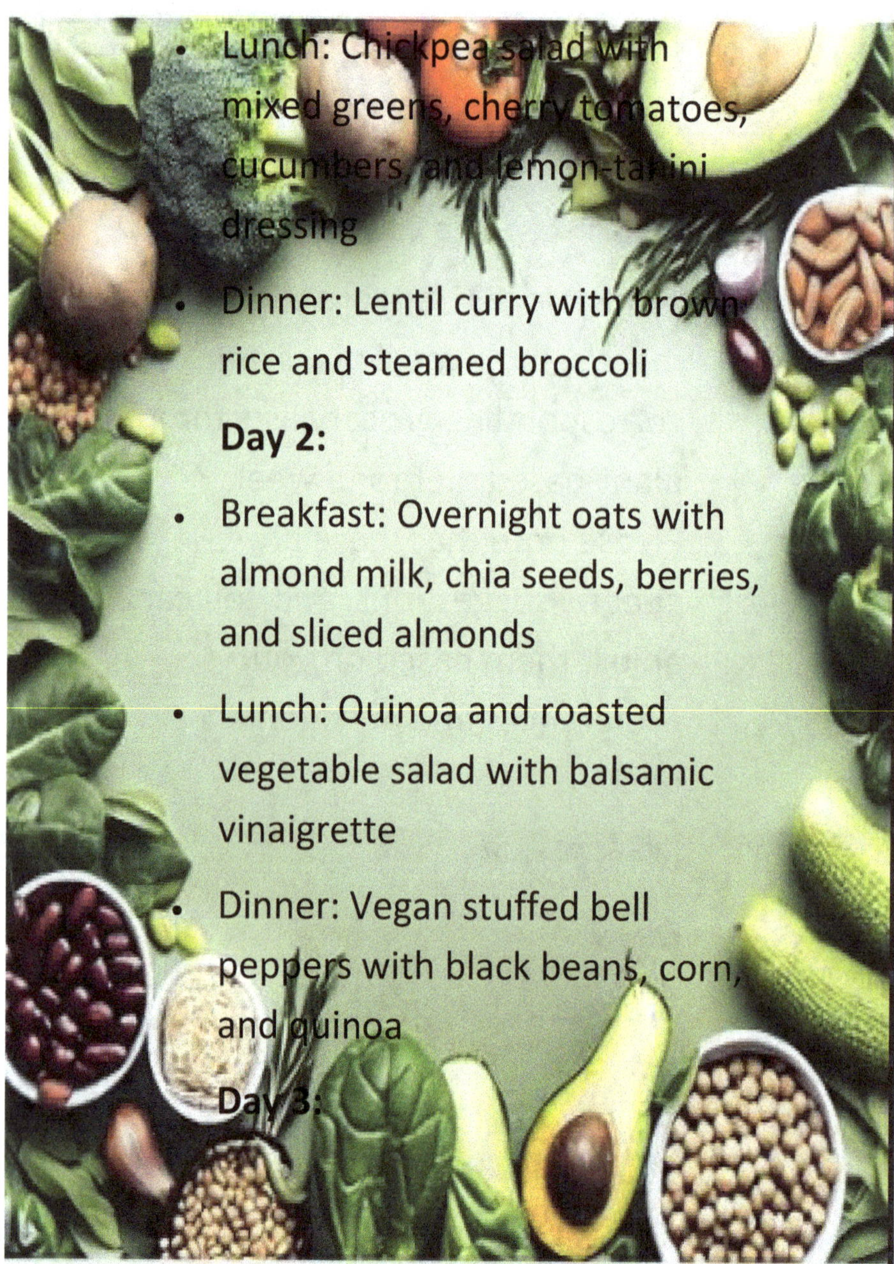

- Lunch: Chickpea salad with mixed greens, cherry tomatoes, cucumbers, and lemon-tahini dressing

- Dinner: Lentil curry with brown rice and steamed broccoli

Day 2:

- Breakfast: Overnight oats with almond milk, chia seeds, berries, and sliced almonds

- Lunch: Quinoa and roasted vegetable salad with balsamic vinaigrette

- Dinner: Vegan stuffed bell peppers with black beans, corn, and quinoa

Day 3:

- Breakfast: Vegan yogurt parfait with granola, mixed berries, and a drizzle of maple syrup

- Lunch: Hummus and veggie wrap (whole-grain tortilla filled with hummus, shredded carrots, cucumber, and lettuce)

- Dinner: Eggplant and mushroom stir-fry with tofu and a side of brown rice

Day 4:

- Breakfast: Avocado toast with sliced tomatoes and a sprinkle of nutritional yeast

- Lunch: Vegan sushi rolls with avocado, cucumber, and pickled ginger

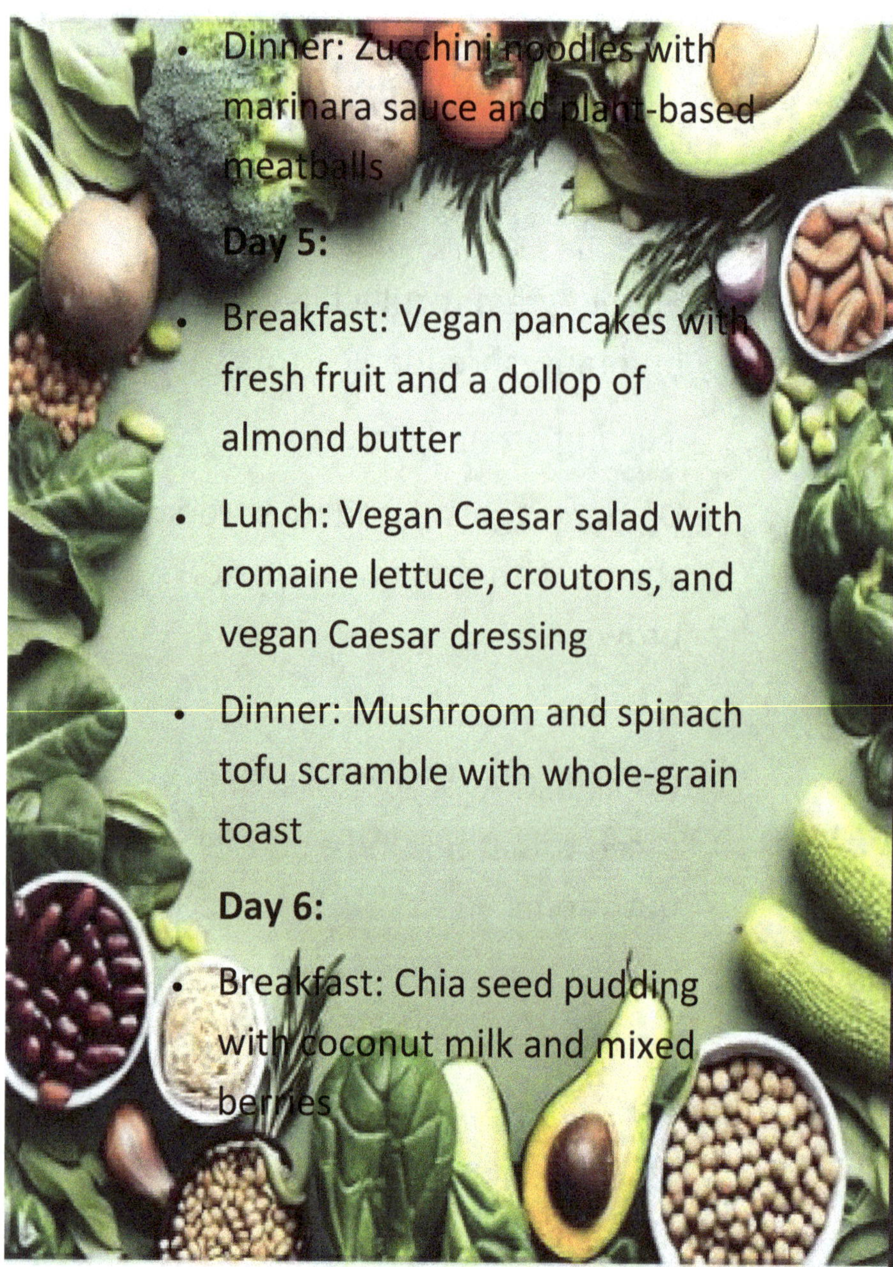

- Dinner: Zucchini noodles with marinara sauce and plant-based meatballs

Day 5:

- Breakfast: Vegan pancakes with fresh fruit and a dollop of almond butter

- Lunch: Vegan Caesar salad with romaine lettuce, croutons, and vegan Caesar dressing

- Dinner: Mushroom and spinach tofu scramble with whole-grain toast

Day 6:

- Breakfast: Chia seed pudding with coconut milk and mixed berries

- Lunch: Sweet potato and black bean tacos with guacamole and salsa

- Dinner: Vegan mushroom stroganoff with whole wheat pasta

Day 7:

- Breakfast: Smoothie bowl topped with granola, sliced banana, and hemp seeds

- Lunch: Lentil and vegetable soup with a side of crusty whole-grain bread

- Dinner: Roasted vegetable quinoa bowl with lemon-tahini dressing

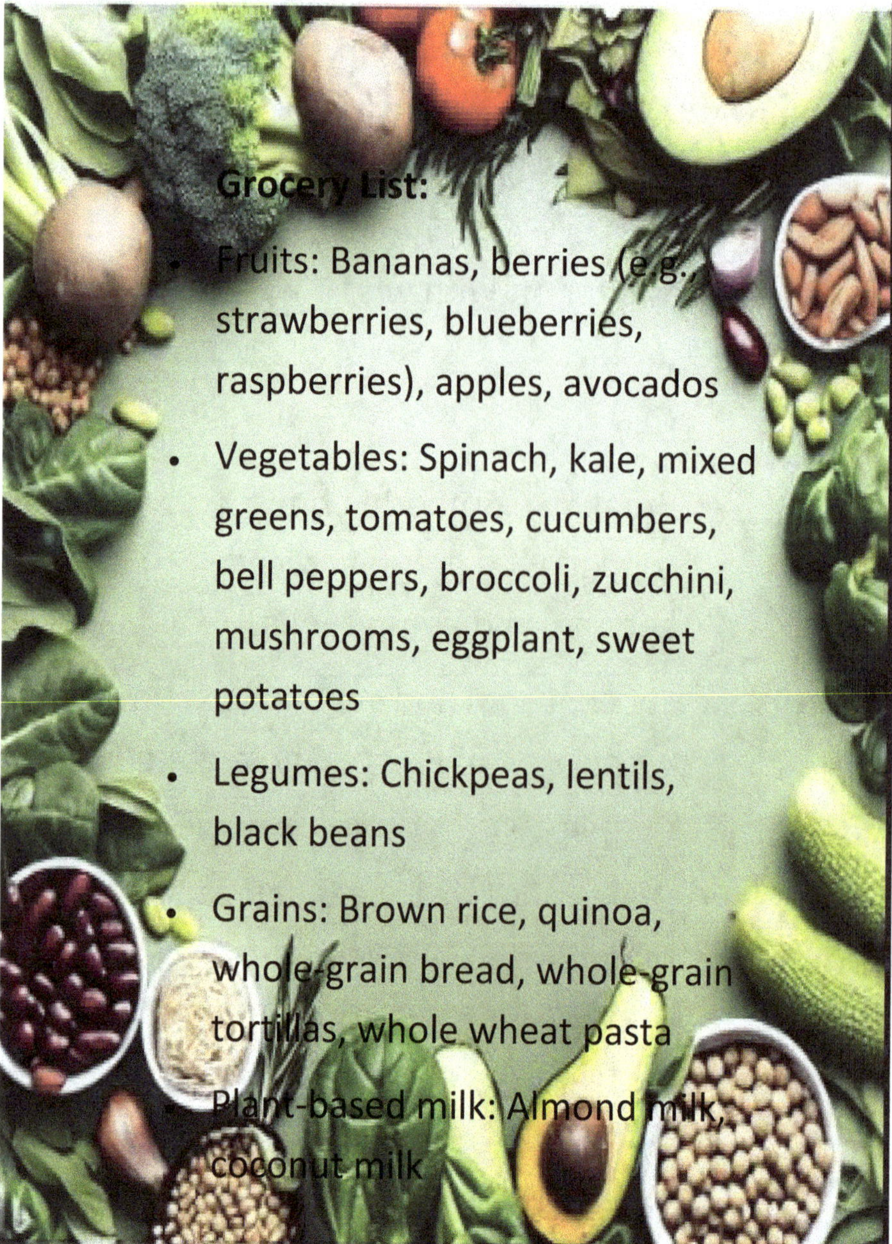

Grocery List:
Fruits: Bananas, berries (e.g. strawberries, blueberries, raspberries), apples, avocados
Vegetables: Spinach, kale, mixed greens, tomatoes, cucumbers, bell peppers, broccoli, zucchini, mushrooms, eggplant, sweet potatoes
Legumes: Chickpeas, lentils, black beans
Grains: Brown rice, quinoa, whole-grain bread, whole-grain tortillas, whole wheat pasta
Plant-based milk: Almond milk, coconut milk

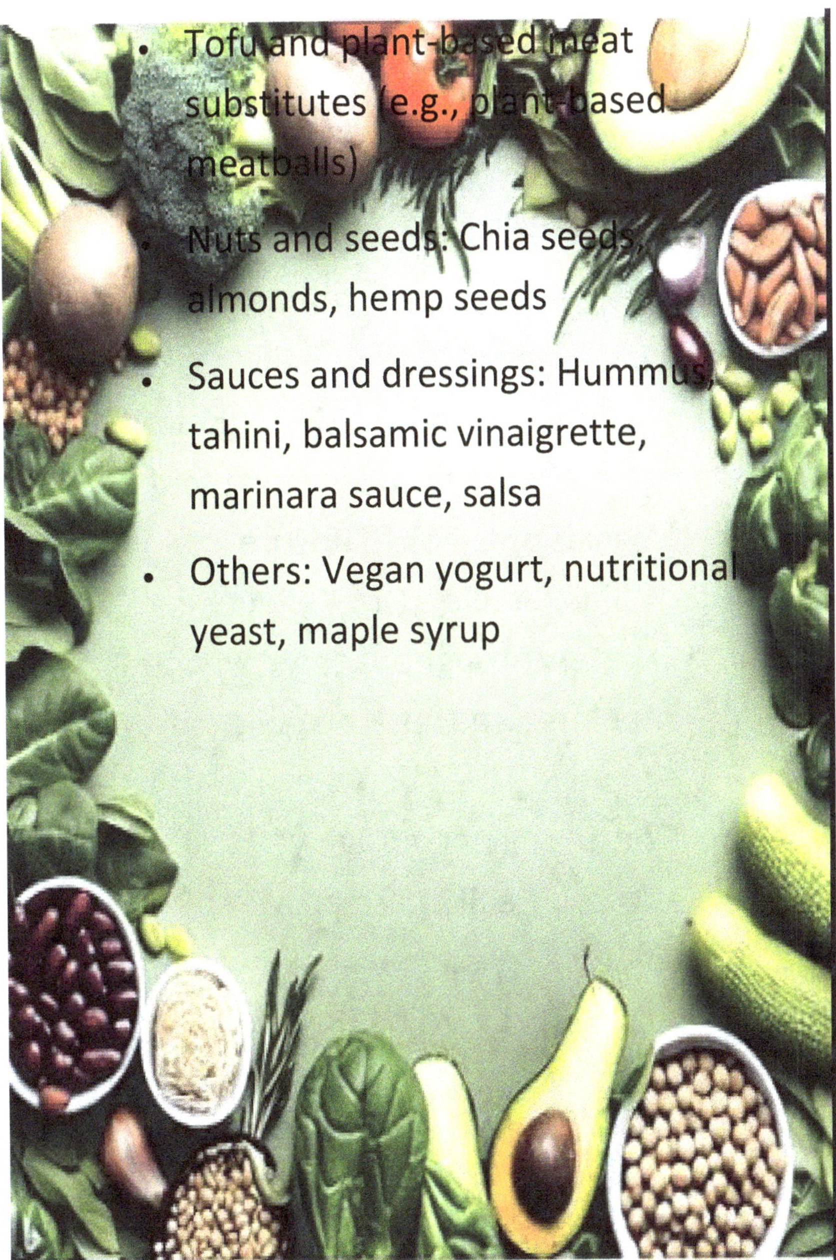

- Tofu and plant-based meat substitutes (e.g., plant-based meatballs)
- Nuts and seeds: Chia seeds, almonds, hemp seeds
- Sauces and dressings: Hummus, tahini, balsamic vinaigrette, marinara sauce, salsa
- Others: Vegan yogurt, nutritional yeast, maple syrup

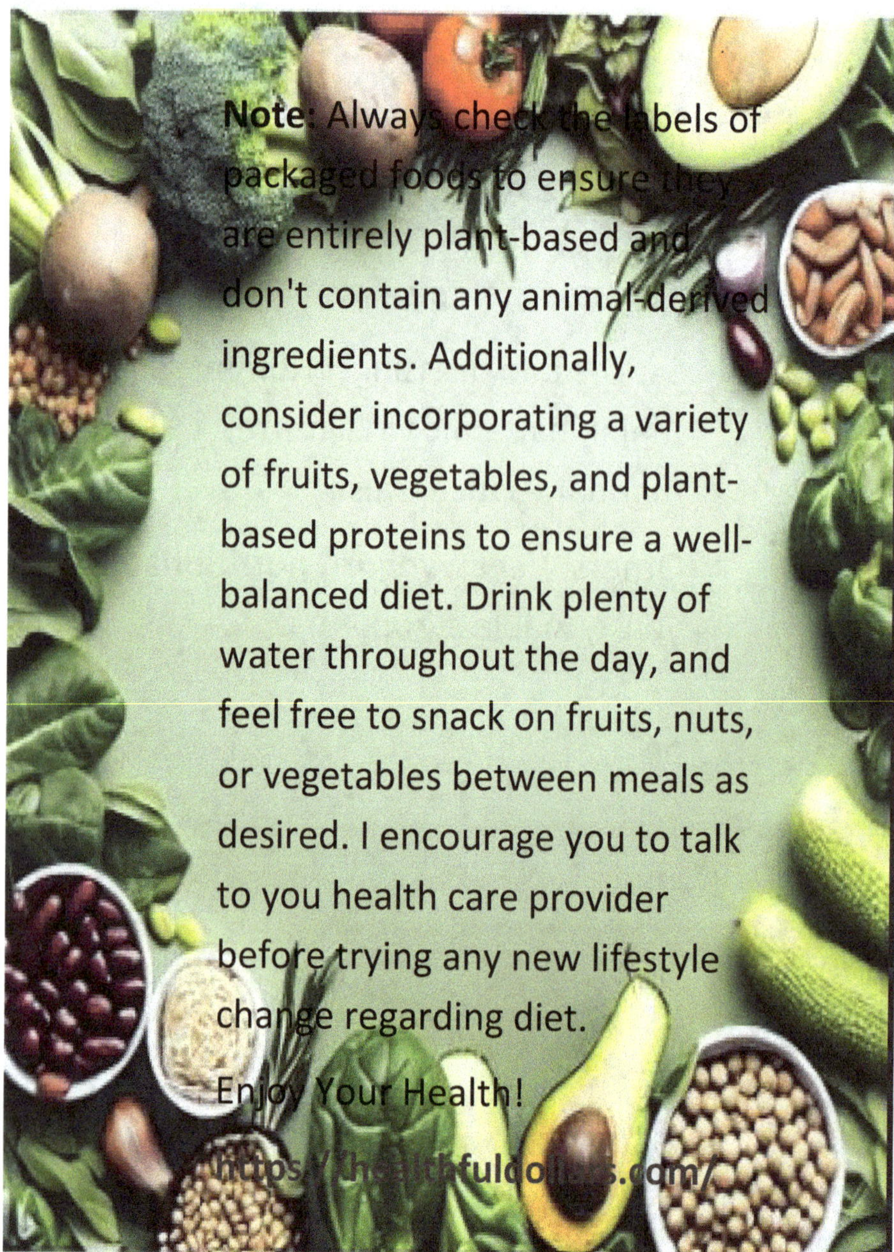
Note: Always check the labels of packaged foods to ensure they are entirely plant-based and don't contain any animal-derived ingredients. Additionally, consider incorporating a variety of fruits, vegetables, and plant-based proteins to ensure a well-balanced diet. Drink plenty of water throughout the day, and feel free to snack on fruits, nuts, or vegetables between meals as desired. I encourage you to talk to you health care provider before trying any new lifestyle change regarding diet.

Enjoy Your Health!

https://thehealthfuldollars.com/

www.ingramcontent.com/pod-product-compliance
Lightning Source LLC
Chambersburg PA
CBHW050740260726
48661CB00001B/323